Bircher-Benner Manuals

Manual for diabetics

Dietary instructions
for the prevention and healing of diabetes,
with recipes,
detailed advice
and a treatment plan
from a medical centre
dedicated to state-of-the-art healing

Dr. med. Andres Bircher
and colleagues of the
Bircher-Benner Medical Centre
Lilli Bircher, Pascal Bircher,
Anne-Cécile Bircher

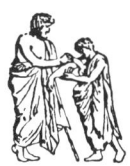

EDITION BIRCHER-BENNER
CH-8784 BRAUNWALD

Bircher-Benner Diätbücher

1. Manual for patients suffering from multiple sclerosis, Parkinson's disease and other neurodegenerative diseases
2. Manual for patients with liver and gall bladder conditions
3. Manual for families and children
4. Manual for fresh juices, raw vegetables and fruit dishes
5. Manual for improvement of the immune system and against susceptibility to infections
6. Manual for mountaineers and athletes
7. Manual for diabetics
8. Manual for support and preventive therapy for lung diseases
9. Enjoy food without table salt
10. Manual for patients with rheumatism and arthritis
11. Manual for men with prostate conditions
12. Manual for patients with kidney and bladder conditions
13. Manual for venous diseases
14. Manual for patients with gastro-intestinal conditions
15. Manual for nutrition during pregnancy and lactation
16. Manual for gynaecological problems and menopause
17. Manual for prevention of cancer and accompanying therapies
18. Manual for headache and migraine
19. Manual for patients with hypertension, cardiovascular disease and arteriosclerosis
20. Manual for overcoming anxiety and depression
21. Manual for patients with skin diseases or sensitive skin
22. Manual for persons suffering from stress
23. Manual for persons suffering from allergies
24. Manual for prevention of dementia and Alzheimer's disease
25. Manual for internal treatment of eye problems
26. Manual for treatment of weight problems, overweight, and anorexia

These manuals are the result of global research, of the development of the art and science of medicine over more than a century, and of the experience of the renowned Bircher-Benner Medical Centre. The reader will benefit from the helpful support of the well-informed physician every step of the way.

16th fully revised edition 2020

All rights reserved, including the right of reproduction in excerpts, photomechanical reproduction and translation
info@bircher-benner.com   www.bicher-benner.com
Book orders: edition@bircher-benner.com

© Copyright by Edition Bircher-Benner, CH 8784 Braunwald
® The trademarks Bircher and Bircher-Benner are protected worldwide
Printed in Germany

The suggestions in this book have been carefully reviewed by the authors and the publisher. However, we cannot assume any guarantee. The authors and the publisher hereby disclaim all liability for personal injury, property damage and any type of financial loss.

Cover design: Kösel Media GmbH, Krugzell
Overall production: Kösel GmbH, Altusried

Inhalt

Preface 9

The nature of diabetes (diabetes mellitus) 11
    The warning signs for diabetes mellitus 11
    The blood glucose level 11
    The standard value of the blood glucose level 12
    Measuring the blood glucose level 13
    The glucose tolerance test (oGTT) 13
    Regulation of the blood glucose level 14

Correction of an excessive glucose level in the blood 15
    Glucose utilisation in the mitochondria of the cells 15

Correction of insufficient blood sugar levels 16
    The effect of stress on the blood glucose level 16
    Sugar excretion in urine 17
    Excretion of ketone bodies in the urine 17

Different types of diabetes mellitus 18

Type 1 diabetes mellitus 19
    The causes of type 1 diabetes 19
    The processes in type 1 diabetes 21
    The clinical symptoms of type 1 diabetes 21

Type 2 diabetes mellitus 23
    Generally accepted partial causes of type 2 diabetes 23
    Genetic risk factors for type 2 diabetes 24
    Other partial causes due to lifestyle 24
    Illness, wound healing, physical stress and lack of movement 24
    Sugar metabolism and arteriosclerosis 24

Glycaemic index and glycaemic charge 26
    The Glycaemic Index (GI) 26
    The glycaemic load (GL) 26

Secondary diseases of diabetes mellitus 27
    The physical damage from sugar 27
    Exogenous glycation 27
    Endogenous glycation 28

Endothelial dysfunction and arteriosclerosis 29

Late consequences of diabetes mellitus in the cardiovascular system 31
    High blood pressure and diabetes 31
    Diabetes and arteriosclerosis 31
    Diabetic foot syndrome 31

Oxidative stress at the centre of the causes of neurodegenerative diseases
and dementia 33

Diabetic polyneuropathy 35

Diabetic retinopathy 36

Diabetic maculopathy 38
    Conventional treatment of retinopathy 38
    Surgical treatment of diabetic retinopathy 38

Diabetic nephropathy 39
    Generally accepted risk factors for diabetic nephropathy 40
    The stages of diabetic nephropathy (according to Mogensen) 41

Gestational diabetes 42
    The following risk factors are generally recognised 42
    Pregnancy with diabetic nephropathy 43

Medical treatment of diabetes mellitus 44
    Insulin therapy 44
    Types of insulin 44
    Methods of insulin injection 45
    Forms of insulin therapy 46

Therapy protocol 47
Insulin therapy at shift work or irregular daily rhythm 47
Inexplicable blood sugar fluctuations 48
Insulin therapy for type 2 diabetes 48
Basal supported oral therapy (BOT) 48
Treatment with the insulin pump 48
The basis-bolus principle 49
The insulin pump with hybrid closed loop system 49
Adjusting the insulin pump 49
Sensor-supported pump therapy (SuP) 50

Treatment of Diabetes type 1 and generally accepted treatment targets 51

Treatment of type 2 diabetes 52
Quitting smoking as part of the basic treatment for diabetes mellitus 52
Diabetes and alcohol 53
Coffee and diabetes mellitus 54

Treatment of type 2 diabetes according to the guidelines of the
Deutsche Gesellschaft for Diabetes 55

Tables for ideal weight 57
The ideal weight of adult men 57
The ideal weight of adult women 58
The problem of food energy 59

Diabetes medicines (antidiabetics), effect and side effects 61
Non-insulinotropic antidiabetics 61
Insulinotropic antidiabetics 62
On insulin therapy in type 2 diabetes 62

Hypoglycaemia 63
Treatment of hypoglycaemia 63

Order therapy for diabetes mellitus 64
Two kinds of food energy 64
The basic regulation system of the soft connective tissue 65
The meaning of food economy 66

The integral law of nutrition	67
Vibrancy of food	67
Secondary plant substances (phytochemicals) with an antidiabetic effect	67
The mineral metabolism in diabetes mellitus	68
Medicinal herbs for treating diabetes	69
The meaning of movement	70
General directives for order therapy for diabetes	71
Regarding the diet	71
Quantity of food	73
Principles of the Bircher-Benner diet and order therapy for diabetics	75
Life order and body training	76
Hygiene	77
Water applications, stimulation of the circulation, air, light and sun	77
Psychological support	78
SHORT SUMMARY	80
Eleven basic rules	80
THE BIRCHER-BENNER Diabetes DIET	82
General information	82
DIET RECIPES FOR DIABETICS	82
General information	82
Bread units and their calculation	82
The carbohydrate unit	83
Sugar in the diet	83
Recipe section	84
Recipes for fresh plant-based foods (raw food)	84
The Bircher müesli	84
Raw vegetables and salads	85
Dressings for raw vegetables and salads	87
Sauerkraut	88
Fresh cereals	89
Fresh juices	90

Plant milk types	90
Hot food	91
Butter, health-food store vegetable fats and oils	91
Soups	92
Soup add-ins	92
Vegetables	96
Salads of cooked vegetables	106
Sandwiches	108
Potato dishes	109
Cereal Dishes	112
Rice dishes	112
Other cereal dishes	114
Sauces	117
Desserts	118
Teas	121
Annex and tables for the diabetes diet	123
Fresh juice day	123
Strict daily schedule	123
MENUS by Season	124
Note on menu design	124
Winter menus	124
Spring menus	125
Summer menus	125
Autumn menus	126
Calculated daily menus for the diabetes diet (1200–2100 K)	127
Table of glycaemic index and glycaemic charge	137
List of recipes	141
Literatur	144
Keyword index	150

Preface

This book is based on vast experience in the treatment of people suffering from diabetes mellitus. Since Dr. med. Maximilian Bircher-Benner discovered the immense healing effect of a strict plant-based fresh-food diet and an orderly lifestyle, the Bircher-Benner Klinik, today called the Bircher-Benner Medical Centre, has healed thousands of people suffering from type 2 diabetes and whose lives were threatened by the numerous secondary diseases and complications. In its typical commercial activity, the pharmaceutical industry is providing us with medicines and sophisticated injection devices for self-injection of insulin produced by genetic engineering. These usually permit partial control of the blood sugar level. However, it is clear from the enormous increase in frequency and prevalence of this disease since the end of World War II that diabetes treatment according to the current paradigm of medical science neither heals nor prevents the disease. The causes of diabetes mellitus and the effects of a "modern" lifestyle and nutrition on the metabolism and the matrix of the soft connective tissue have been thoroughly researched, yet they are barely considered in "modern" diabetes treatment. Medical treatment does not tackle the source. It only fights the symptom: "sugar level". Therefore, the disease turns chronic, appears earlier in life and occurs more frequently. The costs for treatment of diabetes and its consequences comprise 20 % of the total "healthcare costs" in industrialised countries today. Diabetes has become widespread in all areas of western civilisation. It is also referred to as an "epidemic of the 20th century"[1].

In 1980, 153 million people were suffering from diabetes mellitus[2]. In 2013, the number had grown to 382 million, or 8.3 % of the world population[3]. Prognostic estimates have to be continually revised upwards. Only one-third of this increase can be explained by an ageing population, which itself is not due to improved health but mostly to reduced death rates in infancy and to better accident prevention. Only a small contribution is made by life-saving surgeries and medicines. Severe secondary diseases can be delayed slightly by the pharmacological treatment of diabetes mellitus that is common today. Nevertheless, the disease continually progresses until severe consequences occur. This forces us to recognise that the "modern" diabetology has at least partially failed in its task of preventing and healing this disease.

The generally widespread inappropriate diet attacks the fine structures of the soft connective tissue, and the fine capillaries integrated in it, with metabolic slags [translator's note: "slags" are acids and toxins neutralised by minerals and trace elements, and deposited in the body] and inflammation of the intercellular substance. The molecular transport paths are blocked, and the insulin slowly loses its effect on the receptors in the cell membranes. The cells become resistant to insulin while insulin production increases. The islet cells of the pancreas can compensate for this for a long time, until they become exhausted and die. The fine structures of the cells and intercellular spaces and the vascular walls are slowly destroyed. The intercellular substance of the liver fills up with metabolic slags as well. Cholesterol is no longer able to reach the liver cells easily. They incorrectly measure low cholesterol values and increase cholesterol production. The interference with the sugar metabolism leads to high blood pressure and arteriosclerosis. Heart attacks and strokes threaten, as does death of limbs due to occlusions of the arteries in the legs. The fine structures in the eyes are also attacked, eventually leading to blindness from glaucoma, retinopathy and macular degeneration. The fine structures of the nerve sheaths are also affected, causing sensitivity issues and paralysis (diabetic neuropathy). Storage of degenerative proteins (amyloids) causes the capillary loops of the kidneys to thicken until they fail (diabetic nephropathy). Vascular occlusions and depositing of degenerative proteins (amyloids) in the intercellular substance of the brain puts patients with diabetes in danger of developing dementia and Alzheimer's disease early on.

Diabetes is not a single separate disease. It is part of the entire degenerative process of civilisation diseases. Only very rarely does it develop as part of a disease that cannot be healed. Diabetes mellitus, by far the most common type 2, is usually the consequence of a nutrition and lifestyle at odds with the natural condition of our biological system. Starting dietary treatment early enough can reliably prevent and heal diabetes mellitus of the much more common type 2, even where there is a genetic predisposition.

Bircher-Benner's findings have been continually supplemented and reviewed by scientific examinations. They are continually confirmed, in particular very recently.

This book explains carefully and yet comprehensibly the causes and nature of diabetes. It provides the reader with all knowledge needed to let him actively contribute to healing. True healing is not possible without a basic deepening of knowledge about the sense of life, the meaning of diseases, the orders of life, and the relationship to work, society, the self and the people with whom we share our lives. The beginning of this path is the great question of responsibility towards others and oneself. It is a path that will be worth taking, and will be the basis of the path to healing diabetes mellitus. For the treating physician, this book is a great time saver and a valuable aid in guiding and supporting his patients.

Dr. med. Andres Bircher

The nature of diabetes (diabetes mellitus)

Diabetes mellitus means "honey-sweet flow". It refers to the glucose that the kidneys cannot retain because its concentration in the blood (glucose level) has risen too much. The resorption capacity of the kidney ducts is significantly exceeded. The concentration of glucose (blood sugar level) is important for nutrition and the function of all cells in the body, and specifically for the brain. An excessive glucose level will directly damage the tissues, and generally cause metabolic diseases that are described below.

The warning signs for diabetes mellitus

The first warning signs
- General fatigue
- Weight loss
- Increased thirst
- Excessive urine
- Itching, often in the genital area in the case of women

Signs of acute danger
- Drowsiness
- Loss of appetite
- Nausea
- Acetone smell
- Clouding of consciousness

Signs of diabetic complications in the late stage
- Leg cramps after walking for a long time and physical stress
- Blue or pale discolouration of the toes
- Pain in the heart in case of exercise (angina pectoris)
- Repeated abscesses

- Sensory impairment in the limbs, feels like crawling ants
- Feeling of paralysis
- Eyesight problems

Seek medical advice at once if any of these symptoms occur.

The blood glucose level

Blood sugar generally refers to the glucose level in the blood. From antiquity to the modern day, doctors have had to diagnose sugar-containing urine by tasting it. Today, simple test strips and devices are available. Glucose is a very important energy supplier for the body. The brain, the red blood cells and the renal medulla depend on glucose for power production. All other cells in the body acquire their energy from fats as well. Glucose overcomes the blood-brain barrier, directly supplying energy to the brain.

The blood sugar level is normal at first, but after food consumption it rises to abnormal heights before dropping back to its normal level (blood-sugar instability). The urine is still free of sugar. However, sugar may appear in the urine in case of stress, fever or fatigue, or during pregnancy.

After the disease breaks out, the fasting blood sugar level is still normal (albeit slightly or severely increased, depending of the severity of the disease). A small intake of food or glucose stress will cause it to rise to abnormal levels, where it will stay for a long time. The urine will contain little or no glucose if the patient is fasting, but some amount of glucose will be excreted at once after a small carbohydrate intake. The body loses carbohydrates and shows the above symptoms.

The standard value of the blood glucose level[4]

The official standard values depend on intake through food. They are as follows:

Fasting:
3.9–5.5 mmol/l (70–99 mg/dl)

After a meal rich in carbohydrates:
maximal 8.9 mmol/l (max. 160 mg/dl)

2 hours later:
maximal 7.8 mmol/l (max. 140 mg/dl)

These are ideal values. The criteria of the World Health Organisation (WHO) are a little more tolerant. They can be found in the following table:

Assessment of the blood glucose level, diabetes criteria of the WHO

Diabetes criteria according to the classification of the WHO[5]

Normal	< 6.1 mmol/l < 110 mg/dl	< 7.8 mmol/l < 140 mg/dl
Impaired fasting glucose (IFG)	6.1–7.0 mmol/l 110–126 mg/dl	< 7.8 mmol/l < 140 mg/dl
Impaired glucose tolerance (IGT)	< 7.0 mmol/l < 126 mg/dl	7.8–11.1 mmol/l 140–200 mg/dl
Diabetes mellitus	≥ 7.0 mmol/l ≥ 126 mg/dl	≥ 11.1 mmol/l ≥ 200 mg/dl

Criteria for children and adolescents to rule out suspicion of diabetes[6]

Blood sugar control	Healthy sugar metabolism
Fasting blood sugar level	3.6–5.6 mmol/l 65–100 mg/dl
Blood sugar after meals	4.5–7.0 mmol/l 80–126 mg/dl
Blood sugar at night	3.6–5.6 mmol/l 65–100 mg/dl
HbA1c	< 6.05

Guideline for blood sugar levels for adults[7]

Measurement	Regular values	Suspected pre-diabetes	Diabetes
Fasting	< 5.6 mmol/l < 100 mg/dl	5.6 – 7.0 mmol/l 100 – 126 mg/dl	< 7.0 mmol/l < 126 mg/dl
2 hours after eating Capillary:	< 7.8 mmol/l < 140 mg/dl	7.8 – 11.1 mmol/l 140 – 200 mg/dl	< 11.1 mmol/l < 200 mg/dl
Venous:	< 7.0 mmol/l < 120 mg/dl	7.0 – 10.0 mmol/l 120 – 180 mg/dl	< 10.0 mmol/l < 180 mg/dl
Hb A_{1c}	< 6.5 %	6.5 – 7.5 %	< 7.5 %

Saturation of glycohemoglobin (HbA1c) with glucose is indicated in %. It reflects a long-term progress of diabetes of up to three months maximum and therefore represents a sort of "blood sugar memory". Haemoglobin is the red blood colour for the oxygen transport of red blood cells (erythrocytes). They live for three months. The glucose in the blood binds to the haemoglobin molecule and remains bound to it for as long as the red blood cell lives.

The Hb A1c value is lower in pregnancy. It is 5.9 % in most in healthy persons. If it is higher, a glucose tolerance test must be performed. In early pregnancy, the Hb A1c value is uncertain, since it reflects the glucose level of three months, and therefore also considers the blood sugar level before the pregnancy.

Measuring the blood glucose level

The blood sugar level can be determined reliably by the patient with small meters and using capillary blood from the tip of a finger.

There is a method that does not require drawing blood. For this, a sensor taped to the skin displays and stores reliable blood glucose values for two weeks. It is read with a special meter. Then the sensor is replaced. Insulin-dependent patients can use the measured blood sugar levels to calculate the insulin doses to be injected.

There are test strips for measurement in the urine. They also measure the acetone content of the urine.

The glucose tolerance test (oGTT)

This test serves to uncover latent (concealed) diabetes. It is particularly suitable for diagnosis of gestational diabetes or to secure diagnosis in the early stage of the disease.
We distinguish between a simple screening test and the actual diagnostic glucose tolerance test.

The screening test can be performed without fasting at any time of the day. The patient drinks 50 g glucose dissolved in 2 dl water After one hour, the glucose level is determined from the blood plasma. If the glucose concentration is above 135 mg/dl (7.4 mmol/l), there is a suspicion of diabetes and the diagnostic glucose tolerance test is performed.

The diagnostic glucose tolerance test (oGTT) is performed while fasting. Blood is drawn and within three to five minutes the patient drinks 75 g glucose dissolved in 3 dl water. Blood is then drawn 1 – 2 hours afterwards. If at least one of the three glucose levels is above the defined threshold, the diagnosis of diabetes is considered positive:

Glucose thresholds in the diagnostic glucose tolerance test		
Fasting	After 1 hour	After 2 hours
5.1 mmol/l (92 mg/dl)	10 mmol/l (180 mg/dl)	8.5 mmol/l (153 mg/dl)

In early pregnancy, the Hb A1c- value is uncertain, since the glycohemoglobin always reflects the last three months.

Regulation of the blood glucose level

Insufficient glucose levels lead to acute undersupply to all cells, and to impaired consciousness. The most important actors of blood sugar regulation are the hormones from the islet cells of the pancreas: insulin for blood sugar reduction, and glucagon for increasing blood sugar.

The healthy body keeps the glucose concentration in the blood in the standard range at all times by means of the two hormones insulin and glucagon, but also by means of the hormones of the adrenal gland (cortisol and adrenalin). The islet cells of the pancreas contain sensor systems that continually measure the glucose levels.

The pancreas is shot through by nests (islets) of cells that specialise in the production of blood-sugar-regulating hormones (endocrine pancreas).

The pancreas is located behind the stomach, embedded into a C-shaped loop of the duodenum. Although most pancreas cells do not produce a hormone, they do produce important digestive enzymes (exocrine pancreas). They are collected in the excretory duct (ductus pancreaticus) that combines with the bile duct and merges briefly thereafter with the duodenum.

The islet cells (islets of Langerhans) scattered through the tissue of the large pancreas contain four types of hormone-forming cells. Collectively these islet cells are called the endocrine pancreas. The B-cells produce the hormone insulin and discharge it into the blood when the blood sugar level rises. The A-cells produce the hormone glucagon that is needed if the blood sugar level is too low. Apart from this, there are also D-cells. These produce the hormone somatostatin, which inhibits the excretion of insulin as well as that of glucagon, dampening the entire regulation and keeping it under control. The fourth cell type, the PP-cells, produce a peptide (pancreatic polypeptide). Peptides are short-chain proteins.

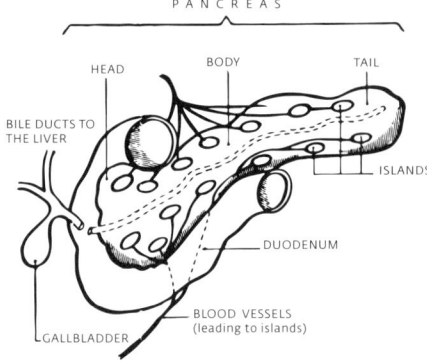

LOCATION OF THE PANCREAS IN THE ABDOMEN

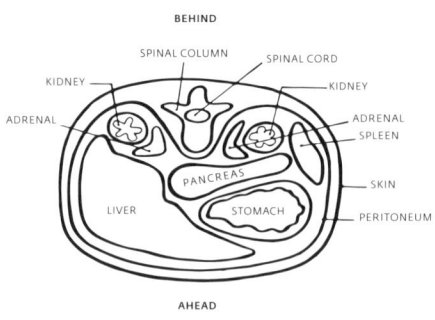

CROSS SECTION THROUGH THE ABDOMINAL ORGANS

Correction of an excessive glucose level in the blood

The hormone *insulin*

The upper limit of the blood glucose level is ensured by the hormone insulin in healthy people. It is formed in the pancreas and discharged into the blood. The walls of all cells in our bodies are surrounded by membranes with very complex structures. They contain many unsaturated fatty acids and are stabilised by cholesterol which is formed in the liver and the intestinal walls. The cholesterol is bound to LDL (low density lipoprotein) for transport through the blood and the intercellular substance to reach all cells in the body.

The cell membranes control what may enter the cells and what is to be secreted from them. They contain special transport systems. For glucose, this is the glucose transport system 4 (GLUT 4), which controls the flow of glucose for cell metabolism. Cell membranes will only let glucose enter the cells under the effect of insulin, while other sugar types, such as fructose, may enter freely even without insulin.

Glucose utilisation in the mitochondria of the cells

The metabolism in the cells (intermediary metabolism) is as ingenious as an extremely complex, gigantic chemical lab in which thousands of chemical reactions run in a precisely controlled manner. Glucose serves to supply energy to this enormous metabolism and provides energy for the cells.

Each healthy cell's cytoplasm contains about 1500 mitochondria, which can be considered the power plants of the cells. If glucose enters these cells, it will enter the mitochondria. There it is broken down step by step until only carbon dioxide and water remain. A large quantity of energy is released during all of these steps. The energy is chemically preserved by adding an additional phosphorus atom to the molecule adenosin diphosphate (ADP), making it adenosin triphosphate (ADP + P = ATP).

Many chemical reactions in our metabolism, and specifically those that serve to build up large molecules, require energy in order to function. Adenosin triphosphate (ATP) supplies this energy by again discharging its third phosphorus atom. Therefore the mitochondria and the continuous presence of glucose effected by insulin are absolutely vital for the formation of ATP molecules in the cells.

Insulin causes glucose to flow into the cells, in particular the liver cells, where insulin activates a number of glucose-consuming reactions (anabolic branch). Indirect activation of the enzyme glycogen synthase (GYS) is especially important. This enzyme causes glucose to be built up into animal starch (glycogen) and stored in that form as a supply for moments of increased demand.

Correction of insufficient blood sugar levels

The hormone *glucagon*

The Alpha-cells (α-cells) of the pancreas produce glucagon. Glucagon is the direct antagonist of insulin. Secreted when the blood sugar levels are too low, glucagon ensures sufficient glucose supply to the cells. It raises the concentration of free fatty acids in the blood if they are too low, and lowers the concentration of amino acids in the blood when those climb too high. Under stress, the sympathicus share of the vegetative nervous system increases the excretion of glucagon via the β-2 receptors. Glucagon generally has the opposite effect of insulin. It ensures a sufficient fasting blood sugar level for the cellular metabolism between meals or when hungry. To this end, it promotes the conversion of glycogen to glucose in the liver (gluconeogenesis), the build-up of glucose from other molecules (gluconeogenesis) and the breaking down of subcutaneous fat, thereby causing the formation of ketone bodies of fatty acids in the liver (β oxidation).

The effect of stress on the blood glucose level

Adrenaline and cortisol

Stress, infections, annoyance, fear or anger causes the brain to activate the stress axis, by excreting the adrenal hormone cortisol via the hypophysis. Activating the sympathetic nervous system by stress on the adrenal gland also directly leads to excretion of adrenalin, which prepares the entire cardiovascular system and breathing for higher performance. Adrenalin, like glucagon, activates the breaking down of glycogen to provide more glucose to the mitochondria, and thus to the cell energy under stress.

In addition, the stress hormone adrenalin activates the enzyme glycogen phosphorylase in the muscles. The stress hormone cortisol also raises the blood sugar level. At the same time, permanent stress activates inflammation mediators (interleukins, interferons and tumour necrosis factors).

Life under permanent stress therefore poses a high additional risk to develop diabetes mellitus. At the same time, it causes general readiness for inflammation via the stress axis, which often leads to rheumatoid pain or fibromyalgia.

Inflammation causes oxidative stress and the formation of free radicals. This increases the risk for degenerative diseases, cancer and dementia. The adenosine monophosphate levels, increased under stress, in the liver and skeletal musculature activate the enzyme glycogen phosphorylase (PYG)[8].

The build-up and degradation of the glucose-storing glycogen are both regulated antagonistically via the phosphorylation of the key enzymes glycogen phosphorylase (PYG) and glycogen synthetase (GYS). This means that storage of glucose can never take place at the same time that glycogen is released.

Sugar excretion in urine

The kidneys resorb nearly all glucose into the blood in healthy people. In case of blood sugar levels above 11.1 mmol/l (200 mg/dl), however, the capacity of the kidney ducts for re-resorption of glucose is exhausted; the higher the blood sugar level climbs, the more glucose is excreted in the urine (diabetes mellitus). This re-resorption capacity of the kidneys differs from person to person. It is usually much lower in pregnant women, so that glucose already appears at lower blood sugar levels in the urine. The sugar content of the urine also inhibits water re-resorption by osmosis. Because of this, the water volume excreted increases if the blood sugar levels are too high. The sugar "draws" water into the urine with it. Consequently, diabetes mellitus leads to increased excretion of urine (polyuria) and increased thirst (polydipsia).

Excretion of ketone bodies in the urine

If there is not enough insulin, the glucose remains in the blood and in the intercellular substance outside of the cells, without being available to the energy-supplying breakdown in the mitochondria inside the cells. The cells remain hungry.

Consequently the body will break down fatty tissues as an emergency regulation, as it would during sustained fasting, in order to acquire the energy it needs. Keto acids are formed when breaking down fats. These are degradation products of fatty acids. The degradation of fatty tissue leaves behind a flood of keto acids, and in particular acetone. Keto acids have a double oxygen tie, so their oxygen atom strongly tries to bind to other molecules. Because oxygen ties mean oxidation, keto acids are strong oxidants. This leads to oxidative stress in the tissues. Oxidative stress means degeneration.

In the face of a drastic lack of insulin, which is more often the case in type 1 diabetes, where the islet cells are destroyed by antibodies, so many keto acids are formed that the over-acidification becomes life-threatening. This is called ketoacidosis, which produces an acetone smell of the entire body that is reminiscent of rotting apples.

To recognise a dangerous over-acidification in time, the test strips for determining glucose levels in the urine also measure the keto bodies.

Type 2 diabetes only rarely comes with a risk of ketoacidosis. If so, it happens only after many years, when the islet cells are entirely exhausted and have mostly been destroyed.

Different types of diabetes mellitus

In 1965, the World Health Organisation (WHO) published recommendations for the classification and diagnosis of diabetes mellitus, in order to clearly distinguish between the different types of diabetes. This classification was changed in 1998, as shown below.

Type 1 diabetes mellitus
Diabetes with absolute insulin deficit due to complete destruction of the insulin-producing beta cells of the pancreas

Type I A: the beta cells are destroyed by autoantibodies
Type I B: the cause for destruction of the beta cells is unknown (idiopathic)

Type 2 diabetes mellitus
In this form of diabetes, the insulin level in the blood is too high (hyperinsulinism) due to insulin resistance. Degenerative slag formation with useless metabolites in the intercellular substance due to poor nutrition prevents glucose from properly reaching the GLUT-4 receptors of the cell membranes. This prevents the flow into the cell. The islet cells can compensate the deficit at the cell membranes for a certain time by increasing their insulin production (hyperinsulinism).

If the condition persists for a longer period, however, the islet cells will be exhausted. Then the insulin level drops, since it is no longer possible to produce enough insulin to supply the cells (type 2 diabetes with reduced insulin level). The WHO classification has the following subtypes.

Type 2 A: without obesity
Type 2 B: with obesity

Other rare types of diabetes:
A: Rare congenital defects of the beta cells of the pancreas
B: Rare genetic defects of insulin effect (receptor defects)
C: Diabetes due to disease or destruction of the pancreas
D: Diabetes due to other hormonal disorders
E: Diabetes caused by toxicity of medicines or by chemicals, drugs or toxins
F: Diabetes during infections
G: Diabetes due to rare immune disorders
H: Congenital diseases associated with diabetes

Type 1 diabetes mellitus

This used to be called juvenile diabetes since it occurred almost exclusively in children and teens. Today adults are also affected, even though the onset is still most frequently between 11 and 13 years of age.

The causes of type 1 diabetes

The cause is considered multifactorial today. Genetic and environmental factors have been identified.

Genetic factors
More than 50 genes have been identified so far. As several of them interact, several genetic changes are required for congenital type 1 diabetes to occur. A single gene is only very rarely the case[9].

In particular the MHC region on the short branch of chromosome 6 could be responsible for type 1 diabetes. The genes HLA-A and HLA-B of this region are of particular importance. They contain the genetic information for formation of proteins on the surface of body cells that serve to distinguish between the body's own cells and external cells.[10]

It is suspected that genes outside of this HLA region have a much lower relevance as a cause of type 1 diabetes. One of them is the gene for production of insulin (INS), and another is the gene CTLA 4 responsible for regulation of the T-lymphocytes.

Environmental factors as cause of type 1 diabetes
It is highly significant that the incidence (frequency) of type 1 diabetes has nearly doubled in industrialised countries in a very short time. This indicates a high relevance of environmental factors such as the lifestyle and diet in the "civilised" countries.

The immunocompetence of the lymph cells, i.e. the precision with which immune cells can distinguish between the body's own and foreign substances, is decisive for the prevention of autoimmune reactions. This risk is always present when an antigen which enters the body is similar to a substance in the body.

The lymph cells are formed in the bone marrow. They then reach the enormous surface of the intestinal mucosa (about 32 m^2). Viewed under the microscope, it is densely shot through with lymph cell nests, like a leopard's spots. These are called Peyer's patches. This is where young lymphocytes go to school to learn to distinguish foreign substances from the body's own tissues. They also learn what to tolerate and what to defend against. The health of the intestinal mucosa, the quality of the mucous layer above the intestinal mucosa cells, the entire milieu in the intestine and the gigantic ecosystem of the bacterial flora inside the intestine are decisive for healthy maturation of the immune cells in these lymph cell nests. Immunocompetent immune cells can develop only in a healthy intestine.

After they have reached immunocompetence, the lymphocytes will migrate into the blood and the lymphatic system of the entire body, where they do their work of mobilising the immune system against anything foreign and harmful. Autoimmune reactions occur in case of an unhealthy milieu in the intestine, i.e. where the immunocompetence of the lymphocytes and dendritic cells is insufficient.

In type 1 diabetes, antibodies formed against foreign proteins also turn against the body's own proteins on the islet cells of the pancreas (i.e. cross-reaction, molecular mimicry). Scientists assume that the immune system for formation of antibodies against islet cells is particularly endangered in the early months of life. After all, it is not fully mature until the age of nine months.

Caesarean section as an essential partial cause of type 1 diabetes
A long-term study on 1650 children[11] showed that the risk of children whose parents have diabetes is twice as high (4.8 %) to develop type 1 diabetes before the age of 12 if they were delivered by Caesarean section, as compared to natural birth (2.2 %). Researchers have explained this difference by showing that Caesarean section, as has been proven in the past, leads to a deficit in the development of the child's intestinal flora. Caesarean section has therefore been determined to be the greatest non-genetic risk for type 1 diabetes. Of course, this has to be considered in combination with other factors[12].

Viruses as a partial cause of type 1 diabetes
Rubella infection during pregnancy will lead to type 1 diabetes in the child in half of all cases. The following viruses are also suspected of causing diabetes: Coxsackie B virus, echo viruses, cytomegalovirus (CMV) and herpes viruses. Researchers of a major international study (TEDDY study), however, concluded that the causative relevance of the viral diseases is rather unlikely[13].

Autoimmune reactions to insulin
Lymphocytes of people with type 1 diabetes react to the peptide hormone insulin. Today this is held responsible mainly for the autoimmune reaction to islet cells.

Bafilomycins from spots on root vegetables that show black rot
Rotting root vegetables such as potatoes, carrots etc. contain special bacteria (streptomycetes) that form bafilomycins. In the animal test, bafilomycin A 1 causes diabetes from documented damage to the islet cells of animals even in traces measured in nanograms. Bafilomycin 1 impaired development of the islets of Langerhans in the pancreas of pregnant mice even at minimal amounts, resulting in babies with type 1 diabetes[14].

Vitamin D deficiency as a partial cause of type 1 diabetes
Consistent administration of vitamin D to infants and children reduces their risk of type 1 diabetes. Children living in altitudes lower than 1200 m, where the sunlight contains nearly no UVB spectrum in winter, are particularly at risk for vitamin-D deficiency. Children with vitamin-D levels in the upper regular range have the lowest risk[15].

Frequent respiratory infections in childhood as a partial cause of type 1 diabetes
Children who had frequent respiratory infections, in particular in infancy, have been found to be at risk for developing type 1 diabetes. Researchers found autoantibodies against islet cells in children as young as 6 months, many years before symptoms occurred[16].

The common general-medicine and paediatric practice for infants is very often an immediate antibiotics treatment, just to

be safe. Yet every antibiotic harms the intestinal flora. In this case the harm occurs before the age of 9 months, when the immune system is not yet fully mature. Likewise, vaccination viruses from multiple vaccinations are applied today in early infancy, when the immune system is still entirely immature. Experienced doctors observe lymph gland swelling and frequent respiratory infections, anginas and otitis media in children after the early multiple vaccinations, which in turn lead to frequent antibiotic treatment.
It is urgent that this practice of the current medical paradigm be questioned and changed.

Cow milk replacement products at short lactation
Infants with a short breastfeeding time who grow up with replacement products made of cow's milk may have a higher risk of developing type 1 diabetes. This is currently under debate[17].

Early gluten exposure and type 1 diabetes
Tests with mice have shown that early exposure to gluten changes the intestinal flora of the animals and reduces their glucose tolerance. It is suspected that early administration of gluten-containing grain will put the child at risk for type 1 diabetes[18].

The processes in type 1 diabetes

As we have seen, type 1 diabetes is usually an autoimmune disease. Autoimmune inflammation (insulitis) destroys the insulin-producing β-cells of the islets of Langerhans in the pancreas. Only when approx. 80–90 % of the β-cells have been destroyed will type 1 diabetes become evident. In the beginning, a small residual amount of insulin can still be measured.

The insulin deficit has the following effect:
As already described, the glucose cannot enter the cells without insulin. Glucose is not available in the mitochondria. The cell falls into a hunger status. In contrast, the glucose level in the blood rises.

Since the liver cells also lack glucose, they produce it uninhibitedly (gluconeogenesis). The liver produces up to 500 g of glucose per day, discharging it into the blood from where it cannot reach the cells. The hunger status of the cells leads to massive breakdown of fatty tissue, so that fatty acids flood the blood. Breaking down fatty acids requires elements from the carbohydrate metabolism that are impossible without glucose. Therefore the fatty acids are broken down via a secondary path by converting them into keto bodies (acetone, *beta*-hydroxybutyric acid, acetic acid). These occur in large amounts and produce a dangerous over-acidification of the body (ketoacidosis). This acid flood impairs all other processes of the metabolism.

After the kidney threshold for resorption of glucose is crossed, sugar begins to be excreted in the urine. This excretion will draw more and more water, leading to a large amount of urine (polyuria) and continuous thirst (polydipsia). If the condition continues, dangerous electrolyte shifts occur and the organism will dry out (dehydration, exsiccosis). If this condition continues, alertness is reduced to unconsciousness (diabetic coma).

The clinical symptoms of type 1 diabetes

Type 1 diabetes may occur suddenly. It is typically accompanied by a massive weight loss within a few days with drying out (exsiccosis), recognisable by standing skin folds and matte mucosa, simultaneous to large amounts of urine. The breath often smells of acetone. Ketoacidosis produces severe nausea and vomiting.

Cramps in the calves often develop due to the electrolyte shifts, and abdominal pain occurs. The patient is always severely exhausted and without energy. They suffer from visual impairment and headache, and have difficulty focusing.

Insulin therapy for type 1 diabetes
These are described in more detail below. In type 1 diabetes, the insulin deficit can always be compensated by the injection of insulin, since the islet cells cannot regenerate. Some patients become gradually resistant to insulin produced by genetic engineering. The complications and late consequences can then be only partially delayed by insulin therapy alone. Therefore the diet and order therapy described in this book is of particular importance for this type of diabetes. Even though insulin injections cannot be avoided, the diet described in this book improves the reaction of the synthetic insulin, reduces insulin demand, compensates the daily profile, and very efficiently targets the complications and late consequences of diabetes mellitus.

Type 2 diabetes mellitus

The former term of "adult diabetes" is no longer in use, since today more and more obese children with poor diets are also affected in industrialised countries.
In this form of diabetes there is insulin from the pancreas. Incorrect nutrition and deposits of degenerative metabolic slags will, however, prevent the insulin from acting sufficiently on the GLUT-4 receptors of the cell membranes (insulin resistance). The β-cells of the islets of Langerhans in the pancreas measure the excessive glucose values and try to compensate for the deficient effect with overproduction over a long period of time. Usually this leads to an increased insulin level for many years (hyperinsulinism), until the islet cells are exhausted and partially die.
Until the 1990s, type 2 diabetes was also called adult-onset diabetes, since it usually occurred at an advanced age. Today young adults and obese children develop type 2 diabetes.

Often type 2 diabetes is recognised and treated much too late, since it develops slowly and gradually. Unfortunately the causes are rarely addressed. Patients may also ignore the issue, since they do not suffer significantly at first. Often health impairment becomes noticeable only after acute, partially irreversible damage has already occurred.

The specialist societies of industrialised countries publish usually consistent national care directives today in the form of decision-making aids for doctors (disease management, integrated care)[19].

Generally accepted partial causes of type 2 diabetes

The cause of type 2 diabetes is considered to be multi-factorial, with obesity officially the main cause. Being overweight from fat, protein and sugar-heavy diet leads to overweight, in particular in the abdominal area around the liver, the pancreas and the abdominal wall. This has been officially accepted as the most important cause of type 2 diabetes.

If a healthy body cell is stimulated with insulin, it will increasingly store glucose transport proteins of type 4 (GLUT 4) in the cell membrane. This capacity is reduced when diabetes is present. The precise mechanism of insulin resistance is officially deemed unclear. It has been proven that this is not a defect of the GLUT 4 transport proteins. The retinol binding protein 4 (RBP-4) is produced in large amounts in the fatty tissue of overweight people. The scope is the same at which insulin resistance is present. Therefore it is suspected that RBP-4 causes muscle and liver cells to react less to insulin[20]. Whether or not this interrelation is relevant has not been determined.

Diet is an important cause of diabetes mellitus not only in obese people. For example, three longitudinal cohort studies show that regular consumption of sweetened, processed fruit juices increases the diabetes risk even in people who are not obese, while regular consumption of fresh fruit – in particular apples, blueberries and grapes – clearly lowers diabetes risk[21].

Genetic risk factors for type 2 diabetes

A multi-genetically caused risk factor for this diabetes form is assumed and held responsible for the different types of progress. One of the genes involved was discovered in 2004. It is called the PTPN1 gene and is located on chromosome 20. This gene is responsible for the production of the protein enzyme tyrosine-phosphatase (N1). Several versions of this gene have been identified. Researchers found the diabetes-risk version of this gene in roughly every third white-skinned American, while approx. 45 % were carrying a form that protected from diabetes and about 20 % of the examined people had a neutral form of the PTPN1 gene. If the protein enzyme tyrosine phosphatase 1 of the most risk version is present in excess, an insulin resistance is more likely to occur. This gene doesn't appear to play any role in African-Americans. Its relevance therefore has not become fully clear.

A large survey broke down the gene sequences (genomes) of 2,000 people. Data suggest that rare mutations in just a few genes were largely irrelevant for type 2 diabetes. The results led to the conclusion that more than 20 genes had to be involved, and that rare mutations cannot play an important role.

Other partial causes due to lifestyle

Stress and type 2 diabetes
Insulin resistance increases the blood sugar level. In response, more glucagon is formed in order to increase the production of glucose in the liver cells (gluconeogenesis). As mentioned, the stress hormones cortisol and adrenalin increase gluconeogenesis.

Mice from stressed fathers often have high blood sugar levels. Stress hormones cause other methyl groups to attach to a gene in the sperm cells of the fathers. This epigenetic mutation leads to uncontrolled sugar production in the liver of the animal offspring[22].

Vitamin D and type 2 diabetes
In 28 studies with nearly 100,000 participants, it was proven that a vitamin D level at the upper standard threshold reduces the diabetes risk by approx. 50 %.
The metabolic syndrome (overweight, hypertension, fat metabolism disorder) was also reduced by half with a high vitamin D level[23].

Lactation and risk of diabetes
A cohort study showed that every year a woman breastfeeds a child reduces her own diabetes risk by approx. 15 %. This effect continues for several years after the end of lactation[24].

Illness, wound healing, physical stress and lack of movement

These are circumstances in which raised concentrations of the enzyme heme oxygenase-1 (HO-1) occur more often. High heme oxygenase1 concentrations further deteriorate the patient's condition, and are suspected of supporting type 2 diabetes.

Sugar metabolism and arteriosclerosis

The effects of a diet rich in refined sugar and quickly digestible carbohydrates (superfine flour) on the fat metabolism, and the increased residual risk of cardiovascular diseases and arteriosclerosis:

Every meal that contains carbohydrates increases the glucose levels in the blood. Carbohydrates are nutrients that are mostly made up of molecules built from hydrocarbon chains. A number of researchers assert that a diet of quickly digestible carbohydrates and sugars plays a large role in the development of arteriosclerosis. The cardiovascular diseases from arteriosclerosis are one of the most important consequences of diabetes mellitus. Many test results confirm that this is particularly often true in the case of processed sugar, white-flour products and other refined carbohydrates in today's widespread excess.

After consumption the starch of white superfine flour is split very quickly into sugar molecules. Sugar types that are made up of different types of sugar molecules (e.g. saccharose in kitchen sugar, fructose and lactose) are immediately broken down into simple sugar molecules, which are converted directly into glucose that is then used to produce energy in the mitochondria. During the process, the glucose is completely broken down into carbon dioxide and water.
Excess carbohydrates not needed for providing energy are converted into fat and stored in the fatty tissue.

We differentiate between simple carbohydrates (e.g. different types of sugar) and complex carbohydrates, whose sugar content is polymerised and bound to many other molecules so that the sugar can be removed only after great effort by the digestive enzymes.

Simple carbohydrates such as processed sugar, white flour products and other refined carbohydrates make decisive contributions to metabolic derailment. Excessive and uselessly supplied nutrients are deposited as degenerated oxidised fats and oxidised (rancid) LDL-cholesterol, organic acids and amyloids (degenerative proteins) in the intercellular substance, also called the matrix or basic substance of the soft connective tissue. This matrix that surrounds all cells of our bodies is slagged with degenerative metabolite waste products – the result of nutrition with simple carbohydrates. Consequently, the matrix is unable to perform its function as a molecular sieve and information transfer system. Arteriosclerosis develops in the arterial walls from these deposits. This can be prevented by ceasing the regular consumption of white flour foods and processed sugar, as well as by choosing whole cereals and natural sweetening sources (fruits, honey).

Glycaemic index and glycaemic charge

Eating food will increase the glucose level in the blood until it drops again by the excretion of insulin and utilisation of the glucose in the cells.

The Glycaemic Index (GI)

The speed, scope and duration at which a food increases the blood glucose level in a healthy person is called the glycaemic index (GI). Figuratively speaking, it corresponds to the area below the gradient of the blood glucose. The glucose content in the food to be tested is calculated to determine the glycaemic index, then the rising curve for a specific amount of the food is measured and compared to that of the same test quantity of pure glucose.
A high glycaemic index means that eating this food will produce a quick, high blood sugar increase that will cause excretion of a large amount of insulin for rapid return of the blood sugar level to the standard value. After ingestion of food with a low glycaemic index, the blood sugar will increase later, more slowly and for longer, a process which will require a much lower amount of insulin. Food with a high glycaemic index, such as the simple sugars, foods of white superfine flour and processed sugar, contain glucose in a readily available form. They have a high glycaemic index and put us at risk for diabetes mellitus and its secondary diseases.

The glycaemic load (GL)

The glycaemic load of a food is calculated by taking its glycaemic index (GI) and multiplying it by its content of pure carbohydrates. Foods with a high glycaemic index and glycaemic load (GL) strongly impair the fat metabolism. They produce an increased blood level of saturated fats (triglyceride level) and a lower HDL cholesterol level[25, 26, 27]. They particularly put us at risk from obesity, diabetes mellitus, cardiovascular diseases and arteriosclerosis. In a study supporting 75,521 women over 10 years, those who ate foods with high glycaemic loads (GL) suffered heart attacks much more often[28]. Heart attacks were even more common in those women who were also obese and in whom insulin resistance had already been documented[29].

Refined superfine flours contain more starch and less dietary fibre, less secondary plant substances and essential oil with polyunsaturated fatty acids. Several comparative studies have shown that an increased ingestion of wholemeal instead of white flour food will effectively lower heart attack risk[30, 31, 32, 33, 34].

Secondary diseases of diabetes mellitus

In 2016, more than 6 million people were suffering from diabetes mellitus in Germany, with 2 out of every 100,000 children and adolescents affected. Among them, 305,000 people under the age of twenty were suffering from type 1 diabetes. If diabetes mellitus is treated in the manner generally common today, it will tragically lead over time to amputations, blindness, cardiovascular diseases, renal failure and haemodialysis. Three-fourths of all diabetics eventually die of heart attack or stroke[35]. According to the health report of the German diabetes association for the World Diabetes Day 2010, the following consequential conditions were diagnosed 11 years or more after the diagnosis of type 2 diabetes. In order of frequency[36]:

Hypertension	80.1 %
Diabetic retinopathy (retinal degeneration)	24.1 %
Diabetic neuropathy (nerve degeneration)	23.0 %
Peripheral vascular disease (PVD)	12.1 %
Heart attack	11.1 %
Diabetic nephropathy with renal insufficiency	9.7 %
Stroke	7.4 %
Diabetic foot syndrome	4.9 %
Amputation of a limb	1.7 %
Blindness	0.6 %

If the diet described in this book is adhered to carefully and consistently, all of these tragic events and complications can be prevented. In type 2 diabetes, insulin resistance, body weight and blood pressure are slowly reduced, while damage in the large and fine vessels and in the nervous system is prevented. Antidiabetic medicines can slowly be reduced and even discontinued over time under careful control if the insulin level has increased, because the pancreas was not too exhausted at the time the dietary treatment was begun. The damage that would be caused otherwise is described below.

The physical damage from sugar

Large quantities of sugar cause important damage from the phenomenon of glycation.

Glycation is a chemical reaction of sugar with proteins, lipids and nucleic acids. It happens spontaneously without any enzyme involvement. This produces advanced glycation end products (AGEs).

Glycation can happen outside the body (exogenous glycation) or inside the body at high blood sugar levels, and in the intercellular substance (endogenous glycation).

Exogenous glycation

Outside our bodies, sugars are bound to other substances when cooking or roasting protein-containing foods together with sugar. This produces flavours and colouring. The food industry uses this specifically to amplify flavour or improve the appearance of a product. The resulting advanced glycation end products (AGEs) used to be considered harmless. More recent examination suggests that they contribute to certain diseases. Glycation outside the organism (exogenous glycation) is also involved in the formation of acrylamide by roasting. Controversy surrounds the potentially carcinogenic effect of acrylamide.

Endogenous glycation

These spontaneous reactions of sugars with endogenous substances occur inside the body, especially in blood circulation. Fructose and galactose (milk, sugar), and to a lesser extent glucose, react uncontrolledly with the endogenous proteins without involvement of enzymes. In the metabolism, this produces substances (AGEs) such as methylglyoxal, 3-deoxyglucone and dicarbonyl. These are stored throughout the body in the sensitive basic substance of the soft connective tissue between the cells, and are enriched in the cellular tissues, where they cause considerable damage. The damage from endogenous glycation, specifically where nutrition contains abundant sugar and white flour foods (i.e. foods with a high glycaemic index), results even without diabetes mellitus, and is even more significant in people with diabetes. Endogenous glycation increases the risk of cardiovascular diseases and arteriosclerosis. Wound healing deteriorates at the same time. Some glycation products (AGEs) resulting from this cause inflammation by binding to special receptors of the monocytes (special defence cells of the blood), thus producing the inflammation mediators interleukin 1 and tumour necrosis factor α, as well as the insulin-like growth factor (insulin-like growth factor-1) and platelet-derived growth factor. This activation significantly increases the risk of blood clots forming in the vessels. Glycation of fats (lipids) in the white nerve substance (myelin) leads to diabetic polyneuropathy and increases the risk of Alzheimer's dementia. The endogenous glycation also increases the risk of osteoporosis, inflammatory rheumatism (polyarthritis), lung emphysema (COPD) and sepsis.

High concentrations of AGEs also result from oxidative stress. This is the focus on the causes of degenerative diseases and is described below in connection with damage to the nervous system.

Haemoglobin A1C results from glycation of haemoglobin in the red blood cells. As described above, it is used diagnostically as "memory" for excessive blood sugar levels over a period of three months, the lifetime of the red blood cells that contain haemoglobin.

Endothelial dysfunction and arteriosclerosis

Endothelial dysfunction results from damage to the inner walls of the vessels due to frequent high blood sugar levels. This happens by reaction of sugar molecules with protein molecules of the inner layer of the blood vessels (endothelium). For a long time, the inner skin of the blood vessels was considered a purely mechanical protective layer and sealing. Thanks to more specific research, it is now known that the endothelium of the vessels regulates the muscle tension of the vascular wall, and thus the width and elasticity of the vessels. The innermost cell layer (endothelium) also suppresses the migration of muscle cells and binds immune cells (adhesion of the monocytes), activates them to form inflammatory mediators and controls their migration from the blood vessels into the intercellular substance and the tissues. The endothelium influences the substance exchange between the blood and intercellular liquids (homeostasis), influences coagulation of the blood and the ability of dissolving clots again (fibrinolysis).

In healthy people, the endothelium of the vessels regulates the vascular resistance as follows.

In the event of oxygen deficit, strong flow-shearing forces and the effect of the neurovegetative neurotransmitter acetylcholine, the endothelium cells produce nitrogen monoxide (NO). Nitrogen monoxide has a severely relaxing effect on the muscle cells. It penetrates the vascular walls to the smooth muscle cells and causes them to go slack. The vascular walls expand and the vascular resistance declines (vasodilatation), causing more blood to flow through the respective vessel.

People with diabetes suffer from endothelial dysfunction, i.e. the regulation capacity of the blood vessels is reduced by a number of impairments in the formation of nitrogen monoxide (NO), so that they cannot go slack. This raises blood pressure.

The phenomenon of glycation and endothelial dysfunction take place in every person who consumes a high amount of white flour and sugar. It is one of the most important causes of the widespread disease "arteriosclerosis", even if no diabetes has occurred. Diabetes mellitus is feared for its vascular compilations. They occur 2–4 times more frequently than in people without diabetes. Increased blood sugar levels (hyperglycaemia) lead to formation of diacylglycol. It activates, among other things, the enzyme protein kinase C (PKC). This enzyme suppresses the formation of nitrogen monoxide (NO), so that the vascular endothelium cannot regulate vessel width anymore. The enzyme PKC also stimulates formation of the substance endothelin-1 (ET-1), which constricts the blood vessels (vasoconstriction). This narrows the vessels and increases the vascular resistance, so that the blood pressure rises and circulation of the organs is noticeably reduced.

The same PKC enzyme also activates the enzyme NADPH oxydase, which forms reactive oxidising substances and free radicals (reactive oxygen species, or ROS). It is therefore involved in the creation of oxidative stress, which is described in detail below. These very strongly oxidising ROS react with the nitrogen monoxide formed at the same time (NO) and convert it to peroxynitrite (ONOO-). Peroxynitrite is a dangerous, extremely oxidising radical that triggers a number of oxidising processes and produces a connective-tissue-like hardening of the vascular walls by depositing collagen fibres, fibronectin and laminin.

The insulin level, which is at least initially increased in type 2 diabetes, and the insulin resistance are also relevant for hardening of the vascular walls and their inability to expand. This leads to a partial interference with the insulin signal path at the cells of the vascular inner walls (endothelium), thereby further reducing their ability to form nitrogen monoxide (NO). Additionally, the insulin resistance promotes the formation of substances that promote arteriosclerosis (plasminogen activator 1 (PAI-1) and ET-1 etc.).

The abundant fatty tissue leads to increased inflammation readiness in the overweight type 2 diabetic, since it excretes adipokines, particularly including the tumour necrosis factor α (TNF-α) which is involved both in the development of insulin resistance and in the reduction of the regulation capacity of the blood vessels (endothelial dysfunction).[37] Hardening of the vascular walls leads to fixated high blood pressure, i.e. it can no longer decrease during sleep and rest, due to the narrowing and stiffness of the vessels.

Late consequences of diabetes mellitus in the cardiovascular system

The AGEs from the exogenous glycation are suspected of playing a role in the development of arteriosclerosis and poor healing in diabetics.

Diabetes harms the large blood vessels (macroangiopathy) by early deposits on and calcification of the vascular walls (arteriosclerosis), angina pectoris, heart attack, occlusions in the leg arteries (peripheral artery occlusive disease, PAOD) and stroke (apoplexy) are possible consequences. Women with type 2 diabetes are at a higher risk for such tragic events than men.

Damage to the small vessels causes microangiopathy. This harms various organs, in particular the retina of the eyes (diabetic retinopathy), the kidneys (diabetic nephropathy) and the nerves (diabetic neuropathy).

High blood pressure and diabetes

People with type 2 diabetes suffer from hypertension roughly three times more often than the average population[38]. From a blood pressure of 115/70 upwards, the risk for heart attack or stroke doubles with every increase of the lower (diastolic) blood pressure value by 10 mmHg. Hypertension results from hardening of the blood vessels in the scope of the endothelial dysfunction described above, which is caused by chemical reactions of the sugar with the vascular walls where high blood sugar levels are often present.

Diabetes and arteriosclerosis

As already explained, diabetics are at a much higher risk for arteriosclerosis than the average population. This also results from the vascular damage described above, which is caused by glycation, oxidative stress and endothelial dysfunction. Oxidative stress from diabetic metabolism causes the LDL cholesterol molecules to oxidise, and these cannot be dissolved by the macrophages. Consequently, they deposit as "foam cells" in the arterial walls. The triglyceride blood level usually increases only in overweight people.

It is very important to observe that all of these consequences can be avoided by the diet described in this book. Glycation and the impaired regulation and hardening of the blood vessels (endothelial dysfunction) normalise, as does the blood pressure and the fat metabolism disorder. It is in this manner that arteriosclerosis and its dangerous long-term consequences (e.g. heart attack, stroke or amputation due to vascular occlusion) can be avoided, in spite of diabetes mellitus. A treatment that pays off. We recommend the Bircher-Benner manual no. 19 for patients with hypertension, cardiovascular disease and arteriosclerosis. It contains important explanations and information on preventing the long-term consequences of diabetes.

Diabetic foot syndrome

About 15 % of people with type 2 diabetes develop painless, badly healing wounds on their feet in the course of their lives, and 4 % develop a new wound every year.

Wounds should usually heal completely within two to three weeks. The glycation end products (AGEs) described above and the impairment of neurovegetative regulation due to polyneuropathy strongly impairs wound healing in diabetes. The wounds often develop unnoticed at pressure points in the shoe, or from hitting the lower leg or foot on something. Such wounds are usually badly infected.

If the nerve damage has progressed, ulcers will develop that may go deep into the bone or the joints (Charcot foot). The bone will then break easily without being felt, since all sensation of pain has been lost. Then there is a risk of continued strain on the broken foot. In that case, one foot will be warm, red, swollen and deformed.

Arterial occlusion is the cause of diabetic foot syndrome in only about 15 % of the cases. Every third patient will show both causes: arterial occlusions and neuropathy.

As a sign of impaired circulation, the feet will be cold, the nails thickened, the skin thin, parchment-like and pale blue. Infections will usually develop that are difficult to heal.

Because of a lack of sensation, temperature and pain sensitivity, damage and injury to the feet often go unobserved and can badly deteriorate.

For such cases we recommend consultation with a podiatrist specialised in diabetes, and the following procedure:

– Check your feet carefully every day for pressure points, swellings or injury, in particular after hikes and when wearing new shoes.
– It is important that you wash your feet carefully in lukewarm water every day, in particular between the toes.
– After washing, the skin should be carefully treated with foot salve with 1 % essential lavender and rose geranium oil.
– The toenails should not be cut with scissors or clippers. Only use a nail file to form them carefully, to avoid injury.
– Shoes should be loose and made of soft leather. Check every day if there are any irregularities.
– Stockings should be of cotton, soft and without seams.
– Due to the lack of temperature sensation, direct sunlight must be avoided and the feet must not be held towards an oven or fireplace to warm them up.
– Do not walk barefoot, because of risk of injury.

Diabetic foot should be treated by the general practitioner or specialised centres.

Oxidative stress at the centre of the causes of neurodegenerative diseases and dementia

These diseases occur much more frequently with diabetes mellitus. Oxidative stress is at the centre of the causes of neurodegenerative diseases and dementia.

Unsuitable nutrition, stimulants and irritants, environmental stress, a disorderly lifestyle, ionising UV-A and electromagnetic radiation and, as we have already seen, frequently high blood sugar levels and glycation all cause the organism to suffer from oxidative stress. This causes a metabolic situation in which an amount exceeding the physiological scale of reactive oxygen compounds (reactive oxygen species, or ROS) occurs. These highly reactive oxidising substances are molecules with at least one unsaturated electron pair, which makes them particularly reactive. They are produced in the mitochondria, the "power plants" of the cells that break down glucose through electron transfer and the enzyme cytochrome P 450-oxidase.
This produces the superoxide anion radical (O_2^-), hydrogen peroxide (H_2O_2), the hydroxide radical (OH*) and nitric oxide (NO*).

Healthy cells can neutralise these highly reactive oxygen compounds by providing neutralising substances. The most important antioxidative substance provided by the body is glutathione, a peptide that it produces from the three amino acids: glutamic acid, cysteine and glycine. Other important antioxidants are ubiquinone (activated coenzyme Q10), vitamins A, C and E, selenium and many secondary plant substances from vegetable food.

In the case of oxidative stress in the metabolism, these reserves have been depleted. Oxidised glutathione can no longer be sufficiently returned to its active, reduced form, since the enzyme glutathione reductase is depleted, as are other detoxification enzymes such as peroxide dismutase and catalase. The highly reactive oxidants (ROS) thus remain in the metabolism, where they can damage large molecules (macro molecules) both inside and outside the cells.

This has dangerous consequences. The unsaturated fatty acids of the cell membranes are oxidised (lipid peroxidation), and this causes the destruction of the mitochondria, exhausting the cells and requiring them to expend considerably more energy to maintain their electrical membrane potentials. Moreover, the lipid-containing myelin sheaths of the fast-conducting nerve fibres in the brain and the spinal cord and in the nerves outside the central nervous system are damaged by lipid peroxidation. There will be further damage to proteins (protein peroxidation) and the hereditary material (DNA peroxidation), which causes the DNA molecules of the hereditary material to split (genetic mutations) and may lead to the conversion of healthy cells into tumour or cancer cells.

Oxidative stress means that the organism is in a premature aging process that will severely reduce life expectancy. Glucose metabolism (in the respiratory chain of the mitochondria) produces water as its end product in the healthy condition. In about 2 % of the cases, errors occur so that, for example, an oxygen atom will connect to one instead of two hydrogen atoms, systematically creating a highly reactive fission product of water, the hydroxyl radical (OH*). This free radical is highly reactive because the oxygen atom of the OH* radical is actively searching for an additional electron from any other molecule. Other radicals include the nitrogen oxide radical (NO*), the chloride radical (CI*) and the bromide radical (Br*).

The importance of free radicals is currently the object of much scientific interest in connection with research into the causes of various neurodegenerative diseases, such as Alzheimer's disease (AD), multiple sclerosis (MS), amyotrophic lateral sclerosis (ALS), Huntington's disease, Parkinson's disease and diabetic neuropathy. Many studies suggest that destruction of the brain stem ganglions by free radicals is a cause of these increasingly common diseases. Multiple sclerosis shows indications of damage to the myelin sheaths from free radicals, so that the immune system reacts against the oxidised lipids. The same happens in diabetic neuropathy.

Scientists today accept that oxidative stress is one of the key causes of neurodegenerative diseases. The process begins with the oxidation of proteins and enzymes, whose spatial structure (tertiary structure) changes and forms an insoluble beta folding sheet structure that is then deposited in the brain in the form of aggregates, Lewy bodies in Parkinson's disease, or ß-amyloid plaques and insoluble TAU proteins in Alzheimer's disease, where they destroy the nerve cells.

Usually the correct folding of the protein is achieved by means of special protein complexes (chaperones). It is suspected that these chaperone complexes are changed by oxidative and nitrosative stress, so that they can no longer perform their function in the production of a correct three-dimensional structure of the proteins. The insoluble degenerative proteins deposited inside and outside the nerve cells cause programmed cell death (apoptosis). Cell death is caused by excessive excretion of the activating neurotransmitter glutamate. Glutamate activates a receptor in the cell membranes (NMDA receptor) that trips a permanent calcium flow into the nerve cells. This activates an enzyme (NO-synthase), which causes the nitric oxide radical (NO*) to form. In the mitochondria, excess calcium inhibits cell respiration, causing massive formation of free radicals (ROS). The radical NO* is further oxidised into the highly reactive peroxynitrite, which together with the other free radicals (ROS) massively damages the membranes by lipid peroxidation. This damage releases cytochrome C, which triggers the biologically specified cascade of cell destruction (apoptosis). The brain has a cell-preserving substance that protects the nerve cells from destruction by apoptosis. This way, they would be protected by healthy adjacent cells. However, since the adjacent cells are also attacked, this protection factor is absent, and cell death spreads throughout the brain tissue. Bircher-Benner manual no. 24 on the prevention of dementia and Alzheimer's disease will teach you much more about the causes of dementia. Manual no. 1 for patients with multiple sclerosis, Parkinson's disease and other neurodegenerative diseases explains the causes, prevention and, to the extent possible, healing of these neurodegenerative diseases.

Diabetic polyneuropathy

Neuropathy means "suffering of many nerves". Diabetes mellitus is the most frequent cause of polyneuropathy. Other widespread causes are regular alcohol consumption, medicines, toxins, autoimmune reactions (Guillain-Barré syndrome), certain infections, chemotherapy and possible side effects of cancer (paraneoplastic syndrome).

Polyneuropathy may have many other causes such as deficits of vitamins B_1, B_{12} or E, autoimmune vasculitis (vascular inflammation by autoimmune reaction), amyloidosis (deposits of degenerative proteins in intercellular substance by widespread poor nutrition), deficit of the trace element copper, heavy metal poisoning from mercury and tin (fish consumption, tooth amalgams, chemicals), lead, thallium (from rat poison), cadmium and arsenic.

Damage to the nerves first becomes evident in the longest nerve pathways (i.e. in the legs). It becomes evident as impaired sensitivity with tingling, a feeling of ants and a burning sensation in the toes. These sensory impairments will slowly move upwards. The motor nerves are affected later, so that the paralysis begins in the feet and slowly moves higher.

The sensitivity impairment is often perceived as "glove or sock shaped". It can be tormenting, especially if the pain is severe and burning. Discomfort from heat, cold or swelling is highly unpleasant for the patients. Since sensitivity to pressure of the body weight on the soles of the feet and for the position of the joints is absent, the gait becomes increasingly insecure (peripherally caused atactic co-ordination issues), making it impossible to walk in the dark or with the eyes closed. Since the nerve fibres of the vegetative nervous system also degenerate, the tissues will be undersupplied with oxygen and nutrients. This leads quickly to ulcers that heal only with great difficulty. Since the ability to sweat is lost (hypohidrosis), the skin becomes very dry.

If the neuropathy develops further, the patients also suffer from problems emptying their intestine and stomach, and from impotence. Later they experience tachycardia at rest and from hypersensitivity to light, i.e. the nerve-related (neurogenic) inability of the pupil to narrow upon incident light.

Your doctor can diagnose polyneuropathy by a careful neurological examination. He will refer you to a neurologist for confirmation with an electroneurogram, and for measurement of the nerve conduction speed.

Diabetic retinopathy

In Europe and North America, diabetes mellitus is the most frequent cause of blindness among people aged 20 to 65. Patients with type 1 diabetes will show the first signs of diabetic retinopathy in the ocular fundus after 10 to 13 years, and 90 % of the patients with type 2 diabetes after 20 years. Moreover, 40 % of patients suffering from type 1 diabetes will develop retinopathy. These are twice as many as those with type 2 diabetes. Retinal disease leads to severe limitation of vision in only 5 % of all patients if diabetes of either type is optimally handled with the generally common treatment[39]. On average, 2 % of diabetics go blind with this disease. Type 2 diabetes is recognised much too late, so that 5 % of patients already have retinopathy when the diagnosis is made[40].

Retinopathy is often noticed very late since there are few initial symptoms. Therefore an annual ophthalmologic examination of every patient with diabetes mellitus is obligatory. If signs of incipient retinopathy appear, follow-up examinations are necessary every three months.

The following risk factors for retinopathy have been accepted: when the disease (diabetes mellitus) begins, and whether the blood sugar level can be controlled successfully. Effective control of the diabetes, so that the glycohemoglobin A1C-level is not increased, can usually prevent retinal diseases. During life phases of hormonal changes (e.g. puberty and pregnancy), people with diabetes suffer from a higher risk of beginning or progressing retinopathy. Other recognised risk factors are hypertension, increased cholesterol and triglyceride levels, or if nephropathy has already developed.

Diabetic retinopathy results from damage caused to the inner layer of the fine vessels of the retina by glycation due to increased blood sugar levels, i.e. by chemical reactions of the sugars with the biochemical structures of the vascular inner layer (endothelium, microangiopathy).

There are various degrees of severity. Non-proliferative retinopathy makes damage to the capillaries of the retina visible, but not its increase and growth. Even the mildest form will show sagging at the capillary walls (microaneurysms). If the damage continues, the capillaries leak (collapse of the blood-retina barrier)[41]. Oxidised blood fats (hard exudates) are deposited in the retina. Occlusions of capillaries lead to pointed or larger bleeding into the retina. The walls of the retina veins may thicken, like strings of beads. If the form of non-proliferative retinopathy progresses even further, there will be more haemorrhages and retinal infarctions from vascular occlusions (cotton-wool spots), fragmentation, thickening and the formation of loops of the retinal veins and zones of the retina that are no longer supplied by blood vessels. The retina swells (retinal oedema) first in individual locations and then diffusely. Growth factors are increasingly released in areas of the retina which no longer have any circulation, stimulating new vessel development (VEGF) in order to save these retinal sections. Thus non-proliferative retinopathy develops into severe proliferative retinopathy within one year in every other patient[42, 43].

New vessel formation develops not only in the retina but also in the vitreous body of the eyes, a condition which massively threatens the patient's vision. The new vessels grow specifically where the optical nerve enters the eye (papilla) and from relatively large vessels of the retina. In particular, during sudden blood pressure increases, bleeding from these larger vessels occurs easily. Bleeding into the vitreous body will cause sudden and drastic reduction of visual acuity. The newly formed vessel branches may scar and shrink later and lift off the retina (tractive retinal detachment). This often causes complete blindness.

The messenger substances for new vessel formation also act on vessels of the iris, causing it to appear reddened (rubeosis iridis). This impairs discharge of the intraocular fluid so that the inner pressure in the eye increases (rubeotic secondary glaucoma).

Half of all people with type 1 diabetes suffer from proliferative retinopathy after 15–20 years, as do 20–30 % of people with type 2 diabetes. This proliferative form occurs frequently in puberty or during pregnancy.

Diabetic maculopathy

If diabetic retinopathy particularly affects the point of sharpest vision (macula retinae), visual acuity is lost, making it impossible to read or drive.
This form of retinopathy also results from damage caused to the vessels by increased sugar content due to direct chemical reactions of sugars in the blood with the vascular walls of the retina (glycation). The blood supply to the macula may be impaired early on. Diabetic macula degeneration is the most frequent cause of severe deterioration of vision in people with diabetes mellitus. It can occur in any stage of the disease.

The diet described in this book, and optimal adjustment of the blood sugar level, may slow retinal diseases or even stop their progress[44].

Conventional treatment of retinopathy

Laser treatment of the retina
This is performed as soon as new vessels form or bleeding in the vitreous body has occurred.
Laser treatment of the entire retina (panretinal laser treatment) applies laser light to the retina on 1000–2000 points in a grid fashion. This causes scarring and thereby preserves vision in the treated points. Side effects may include impaired colour vision and dark vision. Treatment of a large surface will often subsequently restrict the field of vision or lead to new formation of membranes growing over the retina, a condition which impairs vision.

Focal laser coagulation is used to treat maculopathy. Laser radiation scars the newly forming vessels. While this often delays the deterioration of vision, it will never improve it.

Injections into the vitreous body
These are not yet fully established scientifically.
Repeatedly injecting the corticosteroid (cortisol preparation) dexamethasone into the vitreous body may improve macular oedema. However, this may increase the inner pressure of the eye, which may lead to cataracts.
More recently, drugs have been developed that inhibit the formation of new vessels if injected in the eye repeatedly at intervals of one week[45].

Surgical treatment of diabetic retinopathy

Sustained haemorrhage into the vitreous body or retinal detachment with membrane formation can be treated by removing the vitreous body and scraping out the haemorrhage. The vitreous body is then replaced by gas or silicone oil to reattach the retina. It adheres to its substrate thanks to the pressure of the vitreous body. Usually laser treatment is performed at the same time.

Diabetic nephropathy

This damage to the kidneys is also called intercapillary glomerulonephritis, nodular glomerulosclerosis (or diabetic glomerulosclerosis) and, in case of type 1 diabetes, Kimmelstiel-Wilson syndrome. The renal corpuscles (glomeruli) contain capillary coils that excrete primary urine. This is collected in the fine cups of the glomeruli and routed through to the renal pelvis through the kidney ducts and collection tubes.

The capillary loops of the renal corpuscles are very delicate. They are particularly sensitive to the harmful chemical effect, called glycation, of increased blood levels of the sugar types fructose, galactose and glucose on the inner layer of the small blood vessels and capillaries of the kidney, which is called endothelial dysfunction and microangiopathy. This damage slowly destroys the ability of the kidneys to excrete urine (glomerular kidney insufficiency). Diabetic nephropathy occurs relatively late in the course of the diabetic disease. It is often noticed late, after more than 50 % of kidney performance has been lost. Nodular growth and scarring of the connective tissue also occur in the kidneys.

Diabetic nephropathy is the most frequent cause of dialysis treatment in developing countries, where the poorer part of the population has recently adopted the poor nutritional habits of wealthy countries, causing a drastic increase of this disease in the last few years. This is especially the case in India and China, where dialysis is not generally accessible. Poorer people will therefore die of this disease.

Diabetic nephropathy usually only occurs after many years of badly treated diabetes mellitus. It is progressive. Left untreated, it leads to complete kidney failure within 2–3 years.

Homogeneous, transparent (hyaline) deposits of degenerative proteins on the renal corpuscles increase the pressure in them and cause scarring. The glucose chemically adheres to the molecular structures of the intercellular substance (matrix) and the tissue proteins. As we have seen, this is called glycation. These changes activate growth factors, and specifically TGF β (tissue growth factor β) and VEGF (vascular endothelial growth factor)[46]. Inflammation also occurs in the changes due to inflammatory cytokines (interleukin-1α, 6, 18 and TNF α)[47]. The capillary loops of the renal corpuscles determine the filtration of the primary urine. Nephropathy reduces the structural protein of the membranes in the capillaries, so that their filter function is weakened and too much primary urine is excreted at first. The increased glucose levels in the blood increase the glucose transporters GLUT1 in the cells of the renal corpuscles. This leads to increased glucose intake in the cells that produce too much TGF-β (tissue growth factor β). This growth factor causes the renal corpuscles to form too much intercellular substance. The increased glucose levels also inhibit formation of the protein protecting against cell death (protein C), so that more and more renal corpuscles are destroyed.

The earliest sign for beginning diabetic nephropathy is increased excretion of the protein albumin in the urine. The normal amount would be 20 mg/24 hours. Quantities between 30 and 300 mg/day are called microalbuminuria, while more than 300 mg/day are called macroalbuminuria. Microalbuminuria cannot be detected with the generally common urine test strips, but can be detected with micral test strips. A 24-hour urine collection is more precise. It allows the medical lab to determine both the 24-hour-creatinine excretion in the urine and the creatinine-albumin quotient. Creatinine is a metabolite of the muscles. The amount of creatinine that is excreted every day (creatinine clearance) is deemed the measure for kidney excretion performance. When the creatinine value in the blood serum rises above the standard, the excretion of the kidneys is no longer normal, a condition which signals renal insufficiency. If too much albumin from the blood enters the urine every day, and not enough creatinine, renal insufficiency is undoubtedly present due to damage to the capillaries of the renal corpuscles (glomeruli).

Generally accepted risk factors for diabetic nephropathy

Nephropathy does not occur in every person with diabetes. In the USA, every third diabetic will suffer from this long-term consequence in the course of his life. It is more common in some families than in others. This has led to the conclusion that genetic factors are relevant[48]. Several genes were found that are altered in people with diabetic nephropathy. A polymorphism can be found in the carnosinase 1 gene on chromosome 18 (deletion locus q), the adiponectin gene on chromosome 3 (deletion locus q), and the phagocytosis gene and actin-producing cell motility gene on chromosome 7 (deletion locus p). Genetic polymorphism means the occurrence of various versions of a gene. This may be congenital or caused by environmental influences (phenotypical polymorphism). It may develop in the course of one's life (e.g. illness), as in this case because of the massive metabolic disorder and oxidative stress that acts on the genes during diabetes mellitus.

The Carnosine 1 gene is responsible for the production of carnosine. The organism needs carnosine to fight oxidative stress. It reacts with the highly reactive oxidising substances (ROS) and with α-β-unsaturated aldehydes that develop during peroxidation of unsaturated fatty acids of the cell membranes. Carnosine is also involved in the organism's fight against the damage caused by the excessive blood sugar levels of a diabetic, in order to neutralise and intercept the resulting highly reactive toxic, oxidising substances (ROS). Such substances are also called radical captors, or scavengers. Carnosine also can at least partially prevent the harmful chemical spontaneous reactions of sugar with the body's own substances, i.e. glycation[49,50].

Adiponectin, along with leptin and others, is one of the hormones produced by the cells of the fatty tissue in order to inhibit the appetite centre and thus reduce food intake. It also regulates the insulin effect at the cell membranes.
In the event of overweight, this protection regulation will fail, and appetite will continue to be high.

It is noticeable that the genes found are all connected to the fight against oxidative stress. Changes to these genes do not need to be congenital. They may develop because of sustained oxidative stress throughout life, in the scope of the metabolic disorder at diabetes mellitus, and, as we have seen above, due to direct chemical reactions of superfluous sugar with endogenic substances (glycation).

The fact that diabetic nephropathy occurs more frequently in some families than in others does not prove that it is congenital. After all, dietary and lifestyle habits can be similar across several generations of one family[51].

It is possible to prevent development of nephropathy in type 2 diabetes with a diet that prevents excessive sugar levels and that massively relieves the metabolism, and to remedy the insulin resistance. This is another essential sign that it is not genetics, but rather the generally widespread poor diet and insufficient treatment of diabetics, which is the decisive cause of nephropathy.

Oxidative stress not only results from excessive blood sugar levels, but also from:
1) a lifestyle contrary to nature, with a lack of sleep before midnight;
2) the enormous electromagnetic stress today, which can only be partially avoided;
3) a diet containing too much protein, animal fat, coffee and alcohol;
4) excessive cooking;
5) roasted substances; and
6) a severe deficiency of living, natural, plant-based foods with their high content of antioxidative substances and vitamins.

We refer to the dietary part of this book and the manual no. 4 on fresh juices, raw vegetable and fruit dishes.

The stages of diabetic nephropathy (according to Mogensen)

Stage 1
Hyperfiltration. The damage to the inner layer (endothelium) causes the capillaries of the renal corpuscles (glomeruli) to excrete too much primary urine. The albumin excretion and kidney function are still normal.

Stage 2
The more severe damage to the inner wall of the vessels of the renal corpuscles causes the excessive excretion of primary urine to reduce (pseudo normalisation). Albumin excretion and kidney function are still within the standard range but histological examination already shows clear damage.

Stage 3
There is now an additional loss of protein through the kidneys (microalbuminuria).

Stage 4
The protein loss now exceeds 0.5 g albumin per day.

Stage 5
The kidney function is now limited to where regular dialysis treatment is required. On average, this is the case after 25 years of diabetes[52].
In 2002, a new stage classification according to KDOQI was introduced. It is based on kidney function only (glomerular filtration rate).
About one-third of patients do not suffer from albuminuria, even though the kidney function is severely impaired already[53].

Gestational diabetes

Diabetes appears in 6.8 % to 16.3 % of all pregnancies. Where not present beforehand, this is referred to as gestational diabetes, or type 4 diabetes. Gestational diabetes has also become more frequent from year to year. In Germany, it occurs in 13.2 % of all pregnancies. Those younger than 20 experience it in 8 % of all cases, and those older than 45 in more than 26 % of all cases[54].
The sugar metabolism usually normalises again after pregnancy[55]. Only very rarely is this a sign of newly occurring type 1 or 2 diabetes.
A number of hormones that are insulin antagonists are active during pregnancy. They increase the blood sugar level. These include cortisol from the adrenal gland, the oestrogens, progesterone, prolactin and human placental lactogen. Pre-existing insulin resistance is increased by this.

The following risk factors are generally recognised

The risk is increased when there is excessive weight increase during pregnancy (obesity), the pregnant woman is older than 30, more than three miscarriages of unknown cause have occurred, gestational diabetes occurred in an earlier pregnancy, the child's birth weight exceeded 3400 g, there was a case of type 2 diabetes in the family or the glucose tolerance test of the pregnant woman showed increased values.

Gestational diabetes usually does not cause any health complaints. Symptoms may occur, however, such as increased thirst (polydipsia), inflammation of the urinary tract, hypertension and excessive weight gain. The gynaecologist finds changes to the amount of the amniotic fluid or growth impairment of the child. He will perform a glucose tolerance test to confirm the diagnosis.
In some countries, the glucose tolerance test is performed as part of overall pregnancy examinations.

Treatment of gestational diabetes
In 90 % of pregnant women the glucose metabolism can be normalised by:
1) changing the nutrition to wholemeal cereals; 2) avoiding white flour food, sugar, chocolate and sweet, prefabricated drinks; and 3) exercising every day.

This is unsuccessful in 10 % of pregnant women, who will require temporary insulin therapy. Diabetes drugs are not permitted because they may cause malformations in the child[56].

Risks for children from untreated gestational diabetes are considerable
The child is stressed by excessive blood sugar. The pancreas enlarges and produces insulin for the mother too, until birth. Afterwards the mother's sugar will be deficient, putting the child at risk for hypoglycaemia. The child is often born very large and heavy, often in excess of 4500 g, which may make parturition much more difficult. The child is often lethargic or overly excited. If hypoglycaemia is not properly treated after birth, the child may experience seizures.

Children from untreated gestational diabetes are often underfed because the placenta does not form properly. They are then at risk of maturation disorders of the lungs, the liver or other organs. Neonatal jaundice (icterus neonatorum) is frequent. These children have a higher risk of developing the metabolic syndrome later, with obesity, hypertension, diabetes and disorders of the fat metabolism.

The mother is also at risk if gestational diabetes is not treated properly.
It increases the mother's risk of hypertension and pre-eclampsia. Pre-eclampsia is a pregnancy poisoning of the mother with hypertension, protein excretion in the urine and oedemas. Infections of the urinary tract or the vagina are also frequent. Caesarean section is often necessary because the child is too large.

There is a 50 % risk of developing gestational diabetes again in the next pregnancy, though the risk is much lower if the mother is able to breastfeed. Without causative treatment as presented in this book, there is an increased risk of developing type 2 diabetes within the next decade.
Therefore monitoring with the glucose tolerance test and adjustment of the diet are extremely important.

Pregnancy with diabetic nephropathy

This disorder increases the risks for mother and child in all stages. The patient requires multidisciplinary care. In addition to the gynaecologist, a nephrologist and diabetologist must be brought in. If the patient was treated for high blood pressure with an ACE-inhibitor and/or for diabetes with an AT1-antagonist, these medicines increase the child's risk of malformations. They should be discontinued when pregnancy is being considered. If diabetes treatment is necessary, the patient must be treated with insulin while pregnant. Blood pressure is generally reduced using alpha methyldopa or selective β-1 receptor blockers, or in certain cases with dihydralazine.

Gestational diabetes can be remedied with our diet if the patient carefully adheres to it. Oral antidiabetics are not permitted, since they may cause malformations. Insulin therapy is an option only if the diet cannot be adhered to.

Medical treatment of diabetes mellitus

Insulin therapy

Scottish researchers Frederick Grant Banting and Charles Best discovered the insulin hormone in 1921. They isolated it from the pancreas of a dog. Industrial production started in 1923, and since then insulin has saved the lives of innumerable type 1 diabetics. Production by genetically engineered bacteria was begun in 1983.

Treatment by insulin injections is unavoidable for type 1 diabetes. The islet cells of the pancreas are destroyed and cannot produce insulin anymore.

Types of insulin

Various types of insulin have been developed to treat diabetes. They have different effects. Insulin produced from pig or cattle pancreas is still being produced but is difficult to obtain and is usually not covered by statutory health insurance. Human insulin is most commonly used. It is produced by genetically engineered bacteria cultures. The term human insulin therefore only means that it should chemically correspond to human insulin. Insulin allergies and changes to the fatty tissue deposit in the injection points are more frequent in pig and cattle insulin than in genetically engineered insulin.

The strength of the insulin effect is indicated in international units (IE). Insulin U40 contains 40 units (IE) per ml; insulin U100 contains 100 units (IE) per ml. Insulin pumps and insulin pens use insulin U100.

Regular insulin
This is also called old insulin, since its effect profile corresponds to the first insulin that was developed to treat diabetes. Regular insulins act quickly and produce a very fast insulin increase in the blood when injected into a vein. This is very important to treat diabetic coma in hospitals. The dosage is administered with an infusion pump under laboratory controls.

Regular insulin is usually injected under the skin (subcutaneously), as patients can do it on their own. The effect commences after 30 minutes and will peak after 2 hours. The duration of the effect varies between 4 and 6 hours. The higher the applied dose, the longer the effect. Regular insulin must be injected 30 minutes before the meal for its maximum effect to cover the increase of the glucose level due to food (injection-meal interval).

Quick-acting analogue insulins (insulin Lispro and insulin Aspart)
These are chemically changed insulins (modified insulins) that have been genetically engineered.
The effect will occur after 10 minutes, with a maximum effect after 1 hour and a shorter effect of 2 to 3 hours, depending on the dose.
These insulin analogues, as they are called, better imitate the effect profile of the natural insulin from the pancreas. This reduces the glucose increase after eating and keeps the Hb A1C values lower than with regular insulin. This is very important to prevent glycation, endothelial dysfunction of the blood vessels to reduce oxidative stress, and therefore secondary conse-

quences of the disease. Insulin analogues also reduce the number of hypoglycaemias as compared to normal insulin.

Intermediate-acting insulins
In these the effect occurs later than in normal insulin. This is achieved by chemical bonds to protamine, zinc, surfen or by using proinsulin that will only slowly be converted to effective insulin. Intermediate-acting insulins must be injected subcutaneously.
Intermediate-acting insulins are used for the conventional and intensified conventional insulin therapy as described below, and if insulin therapy is combined with oral antidiabetics (diabetes tablets).

NPH insulins (neutral protamine Hagedorn insulins, intermediate-acting insulins)
NPH insulins have a delayed effect that lasts longer than regular insulin. This is achieved by chemically binding regular insulin to protamine.
The effect of the NPH insulins starts after 2 hours and peaks after 6 hours. Its effective duration is 8 to 12 hours, depending on insulin dose.
NPH insulin serves to cover the basic insulin demand of the organism.

Mixed insulins
NPH insulin can be mixed with regular insulin or rapidly acting insulin analogues. This way, a short and a medium insulin effect are combined. Mixed insulins are particularly suitable for treatment according to the pattern of conventional insulin therapy, with two or three insulin injections per day. This reduces the number of necessary injections, and the insulin profile is to some degree adjusted to the metabolic demand.

Lente insulins, zinc-delayed insulins
In these insulins, regular insulin is chemically bound with zinc, giving them the form of a crystalline suspension. Lente insulins are also injected subcutaneously.

However, these crystalline suspensions can be absorbed by the body very differently. The effect is not satisfactorily secure, and lasts for 12 to 24 hours. The long effect duration limits the patients, since hypoglycaemia is likely during physical activity and at night.

Semilente insulins
This insulin is also zinc-delayed. The effect occurs earlier than in NPH insulins. It begins after 90 minutes, peaks after 5 to 10 hours, and lasts up to 16 hours. Semilente insulin can be used when high blood sugar levels were measured during the second half of the night (i.e. early morning) under intermediate-acting insulin (NPH insulin).

Surfen insulins
These delayed insulins used to be common. The effect was delayed by chemically bonding regular insulin to surfen, which is from synthetic urea. These insulins caused reduction of the subcutaneous fatty tissue in the injection area (lipodystrophy, lipoatrophy), which is the main reason surfen insulins are not often used anymore.

The long-acting analogue insulin glargine
The effect of this new insulin type is 16 to 30 hours, depending on the dose, with the benefit that one injection per day is sufficient. The effect profile is more consistent than that of NPH insulin, meaning that the peak is relatively flat and the insulin level at night is not as high. This reduces the risk of hypoglycaemia at night, as compared to NPH insulin. It is used mainly for patients who tend to develop hypoglycaemia at night.

Methods of insulin injection

Insulin must be injected in the subcutaneous fat tissue, either by means of a disposable syringe (or a practical insulin pen) or continually with an insulin pump. Intrave-

nous or intramuscular insulin injections by the doctor are rarely necessary. Injecting insulin in the same place several times will cause the fatty tissue there to grow (lipohypertrophy). Therefore, the injection point must be changed at every injection.
Type 1 diabetes requires injection of a long-acting insulin in the morning to cover the basic demand, and a short-acting insulin for the main meals.

Disposable insulin syringes
Disposable insulin syringes with very fine needles are available today. They are found in trade, in particular as emergency equipment. Disposable syringes with insulin U40 contain 40 units of insulin per ml. Insulin U100 prepared syringes contain 100 units/ml. Children and very slim adults use needles that are 4–6 mm long; otherwise, syringes with needles 8, 10 or 12 mm long are used.

The insulin pen
It looks like a slightly bulky ballpoint pen and can be equipped with an insulin cartridge. A rotating wheel is used to adjust the desired insulin dose, then the stroke button is pushed, which pushes the piston in the syringe cylinder forward to where the set dose of insulin will be injected. Insulin cartridges are available in different sizes. The most frequent one holds 3 ml insulin U100. One ml contains 100 units of insulin.

The associated needles are pointed on both sides to reduce injury as much as possible. They have a plastic thread to screw them onto the front of the pen. The backpoint of the needle punctures the rubber membrane of the cartridge. Each needle is only used once. There are various needle lengths that can be chosen on the basis of the thickness of the layer of fat of the subcutaneous tissue. There are also disposable pens that are fully equipped.

Forms of insulin therapy

Various forms of treatment have been developed in order to meet the special situation of each patient.

Conventional insulin therapy (CT)
This traditional injection therapy is suitable for people with type 2 diabetes and an already reduced insulin level. In this case, the pancreas is so exhausted that improvement of the metabolism by dietary treatment and additional medication is no longer sufficient. The disease will only reach this stage in the later course, after insufficient treatment of diabetes. This type of insulin therapy requires great discipline in compliance with the diet and a fixed daily schedule. For conventional insulin therapy the insulin is injected at fixed times of the day, at a fixed dose.

Intensified conventional insulin therapy (ICT)
ICT means that long-acting insulin is injected in the morning, and an insulin bolus is added for every meal (basis-bolus treatment). In medical terms, a bolus is a specific, measured amount. This method is suitable for type 1 diabetes and for type 2 diabetics whose pancreas is so exhausted that it can produce very little insulin. The body needs a certain amount of insulin even when not eating. Depending on the insulin chosen, one to three injections per day will be needed.

The bolus injections cover the blood sugar increase from the meals. The bolus is injected in addition to the meals, as well as in case of hyperglycaemia. The number of units of the basic injections must be adjusted to correspond to the expected physical stress of the day.
ICT permits a more flexible solution than CT, and is better at imitating the natural insulin secretion of the pancreas.

Functional insulin therapy (FIT)
This treatment method has refined the ICT method to better imitate the effect of the pancreas. It is particularly suitable for children, teens and younger adults with type 1 diabetes. Children and their parents are trained in group courses at the university hospital. Meals are skipped deliberately to determine the individual daily demand of long-acting basal insulin without glucose supply through food (basal dose). The patient calculates the insulin demand for the meal bolus on the basis of the glycaemic index and the amount of the food that he plans to eat. Tables for the glycaemic index are available in dietary counselling and can be downloaded from the internet. Functional insulin therapy (FIT) has the advantage of allowing greater flexibility in daily schedules, and thus more freedom is planning meal times. The disadvantage is that a more insulin injections are needed per day.

Supplementary insulin therapy (SIT)
This is chosen for people with type 2 diabetes whose pancreas is not yet exhausted and is thus able to generate high insulin levels. However, these levels are insufficiently effective because of insulin resistance caused by poor nutrition. Although these patients are usually treated with metformin, their blood sugar levels remain too high, especially after meals. Glycohemoglobin A1C in particular is too high, so the patients are greatly endangered by tragic secondary diseases and complications. During SIT, the patients inject an insulin bolus with every meal. This is only a temporary emergency solution and will no longer be necessary with the diet described in this book. Under these conditions it will soon be possible to discontinue the insulin bolus injections and, a little later, the metformin, under medical control.

Therapy protocol

All factors that influence blood sugar should be noted in insulin therapy. This is necessary for calculating the insulin dose.

Every blood sugar measurement, its time of day and whether it took place before or after a meal must be recorded. The food taken in and the carbohydrate content are recorded. Also, events that lower the blood sugar level and thus require less insulin (e.g. physical work, strenuous efforts, intensive movement and sports) are recorded, as are events which increase the blood sugar level (e.g. sweating and stress).

This protocol is best kept in a separate booklet or a specially programmed electronic device (diabetes management software).
This programme is now included in most blood pressure devices. They automatically record the blood sugar values and their times. You can also enter additional information in the programme. An interface cable connected to a computer makes it possible to send this information to the doctor by email if an emergency has occurred, and if consultation on the phone is required.

Insulin therapy at shift work or irregular daily rhythm

Shift work will cause sleeping issues sooner or later. The body will become up to 40 % more sensitive to insulin. Shift changes also cause hormonal issues so that excessive blood sugar values often result in the morning or evening.

A diabetic should do anything he can to replace shift work by regular working hours. A doctor may help with this.

Inexplicable blood sugar fluctuations

Most fluctuations are easily explained. However, among people with type 1 diabetes there are some who may suffer severe, inexplicable blood sugar fluctuations so that insulin therapy is difficult to adjust. This phenomenon, called "brittle diabetes", can be explained by the remaining (and strongly fluctuating) insulin production of the pancreas. At the beginning of insulin therapy for type 1 diabetes, insulin demand can suddenly drop because the pancreas has increased insulin production again. This is explained by immunological phenomena on the islet cells that may occur in the scope of the autoimmune processes that destroy them, called "diabetes honeymoon".

Insulin therapy for type 2 diabetes

In type 2 diabetes, insulin therapy is required only at a very late stage, and only if treatment was insufficient so that the insulin level the pancreas can still produce has already dropped significantly because the islet cells are completely exhausted and have partially died.
Treating people with type 2 diabetes with insulin will often reduce their weight and increase their insulin resistance. As long as the islet cells of the pancreas are not entirely exhausted (so that the insulin level is still clearly increased), type 2 diabetes can be reliably healed with the diet described in this book and under medical control. This way insulin therapy and medical treatment, with their risks of multiple side effects and hypoglycaemias, can be avoided.

Basal supported oral therapy (BOT)

Sometimes, doctors will recommend "basal supported oral therapy" (BOT) in type 2 diabetes if excessive fasting blood sugar values are measured in the early morning under oral antidiabetics. BOT means that long-acting insulin is injected as basal insulin in the evening, in order to cover the sugar formation in the liver (gluconeogenesis) at night.

Treatment with the insulin pump

An insulin pump is a small medical device for continuous subcutaneous insulin infusion (CSII). Introducing insulin uninterrupted in the subcutaneous tissue requires a catheter, i.e. a needle (cannula), which are available in various lengths, with a small tube. The needle can be injected into the subcutaneous tissue by the patient after thorough disinfection. The needle has a self-adhesive patch through which the tube (catheter) is routed out. This is taped tightly to the skin above the injection point. The tube is screwed to the insulin pump. The insulin pump is about matchbox sized, and can be attached to a belt.
Every 3 days, a new sterile infusion set with a new cannula must be placed in a new location in order to avoid infection and to prevent the subcutaneous fat from enlarging under the insulin effect (lipohypertrophy). There are steel and Teflon cannulas, if steel cannulas are not tolerated. Most insulin pumps have a Luer-Lock connection that can be screwed on to connect the catheter to the pump. If it does not fit the pump, connection pieces (adapters) are available (Luer P500S or 700 S).

Unfortunately the insulin pump in its current state of technology cannot replace a healthy pancreas, since it cannot continually measure glucose concentration. There are insulin pumps with an integrated blood sugar measuring system, but they cannot determine automatically how much insulin to discharge. The insulin demand also depends on many external factors, such as stress, physical work and movement. Although it is still necessary to determine the blood sugar several times per day with an insulin pump, many diabetics can live almost like healthy people with them.

The basis-bolus principle

The insulin pump can be set to a basal rate that covers the basic demand for insulin, as well as individually chosen boluses (injection volumes are measured for meals and to correct glucose levels). This is called the basal-bolus principle. The pump contains a reservoir with one insulin type, either regular insulin or rapidly acting analogue insulin. In some pump models, the reservoir is small and cylindrical. It is filled sterile with a piston similar to an injection syringe. Other models use a complete insulin ampoule similar to the one inserted into a pen. An insulin reservoir in a pump contains between 1.5 and 3 ml insulin U100 (at 100 units per ml), and can discharge 150 to 300 insulin units as a result.

The insulin pump is a good alternative for ICT therapy in type 1 diabetes, with the benefit that the meal bolus can be adjusted to the meal that is eaten.
In contrast to ICT therapy, where the insulin effect is irregular over time, the insulin pump discharges a rapidly acting insulin approximately every 3 minutes, thereby producing a balanced basic insulin level that only needs to be adjusted by setting the bolus injections for meals and physical activity.

The insulin pump must be adjusted in a specialised clinic or hospital. The diabetologist will calculate the individual basic demand and adjust for it and the bolus doses. He will explain to the patient how to operate the pump and how to adjust the bolus dosages to meals, as well as how to set pump breaks, e.g. during hard physical activity. He will also show the patient how to ensure sterility and how to replace the catheter.

The insulin pump with hybrid closed loop system

Since 2016, this pump model has been approved for treating teens 14 years and up and adults. Its safety for patients has been proven. This pump model is also called an "artificial pancreas". The patient does not have to measure blood sugar or inject insulin.
The MiniMed 670 model by Medtron measures the glucose concentration in the tissue fluids at the site of the probe every five minutes and adjusts the insulin dose to the current need.
Nevertheless, strongly increased insulin demands for carbohydrate-rich meals must be adjusted by the patient.
The device is not suitable for children or people who need fewer than eight insulin units per day[57].

Adjusting the insulin pump

Current insulin pumps offer the following functions:
The "multiple basal rate programming" function permits adjustment of the five-minute discharge of the insulin basal rates to the current demand at any time during the day or night.

The "basal rate profile" function permits choosing a day profile that corresponds to the current individual demand. The profile for insulin demand in the course of a day may vary considerably, depending on the patient. This function adjusts the day profile to the changed insulin demand due to physical exercise on work days or for training and sports, as well as to changed demands on weekends, shift work or travel.

The "bolus option" function adjusts the speed of insulin bolus discharge during a meal on the basis of the glycaemic index of the food eaten.

The "bolus calculator" function can be used to calculate the size of the bolus on the basis of the currently measured blood sugar level, the target glucose level and the insulin sensitivity.

Some insulin pumps offer the option of connecting a blood sugar meter and a remote control for setting the size of the bolus without having to take the device from its holder.

Sensor-supported pump therapy (SuP)

On these devices, a sensor can be connected that continually communicates the glucose concentration in the tissue fluid to the probe in the pump. If the sensor measures insufficient glucose values, the pump will automatically interrupt the insulin supply on a temporary basis.

Treatment of Diabetes type 1 and generally accepted treatment targets[58, 59]

Type 1 diabetes must be treated with insulin immediately after diagnosis. The pancreas is then very likely hormone-inactive. Delays are not permitted, since diabetic coma may occur within just a few hours. It is better to start treatment in a hospital where proper supervision and immediate training are available.

This form of diabetes often starts early in life. The risk of secondary diseases is therefore high. It is particularly important to avoid high blood sugar values, even after meals, as glycation causes vascular damage (angiopathy) of the eyes, kidneys and entire body, and damages the brain and nerves, causing polyneuropathy and dementia. The diet described in this book is particularly important for type 1 diabetes. It reduces the insulin demand considerably and balances it throughout the day, thereby more effectively preventing dangerous blood sugar peaks after meals and hypoglycaemias.

As a target, at least half of all blood sugar values measured should be in the range of 4.4 to 6.7 mmol/l (80–120 mg/dl). The content of glycohemoglobin (HbA1C) must be as low as it can be without causing hypoglycaemia. This is possible if the profile of insulin injections is as balanced as possible and adjusted to individual demand. It is best performed by injection according to intensified or functional insulin therapy, or with an insulin pump, and by avoiding blood sugar peaks using the diet as described in this book. For HbA1C values above 7.5%, there is a high risk of consequential damage and complications of diabetes.

Regime for intensified insulin therapy

Intensified insulin therapy	
Breakfast	Regular insulin or short-acting analogue insulin (poss. plus a long-acting insulin)
Lunch	Regular insulin or short-acting analogue insulin
Dinner	Regular insulin or short-acting analogue insulin
Night	NPH-insulin (long-acting human insulin) or a long-acting analogue insulin

Sometimes further injections with basal insulin are needed to balance out the effect profile. If one wishes to eat in the afternoon, interim injection of the short-acting or analogue insulin is necessary. During training, the patients learn to adjust the dose for the short-acting insulin according to the carbohydrate units (called bread units) that they eat. They will learn to reduce their insulin dose under physical exercise and to increase the dose slightly if ill, e.g. when they have a cold.

Treatment of type 2 diabetes

Insulin resistance can be improved by losing weight and moving more. This reliably reduces the blood sugar level and insulin demand, which both occur more strongly and quickly than the adjustment of blood pressure. Reducing weight by 10 kg will lead to a normal fasting blood sugar level in half of all patients. Unfortunately, this improvement will not last if the weight reduction was achieved only by reducing calories. Most patients are unable to maintain their lower body weight. Widespread dietary advice does not pervasively change diet and lifestyle, nor is the metabolic interference that causes obesity and diabetes removed. Given this experience of unsuccessful long-term weight reduction, medicine currently favours early treatment with medication. If weight reduction is impossible, surgical bridging of the stomach and the upper small intestine (ADIB, antidiabetic bypass)[60] is recommended. However, this leads to massive side effects and problems.

The meaning of movement and hiking in diabetes mellitus

Physical exercise causes more glucose to enter the muscle cells. Stressing muscles for more than half an hour will additionally supply them with fats from the fat tissue. The muscle cells will also grow more sensitive to insulins. Therefore, the blood sugar level drops due to muscle work if the insulin dose is not increased, while the metabolic performance of the muscles increases. Hiking every day will reduce the fat in the abdominal cavity, the abdominal wall, the buttocks and the thighs. Other risk factors for cardiovascular diseases and secondary diseases of diabetes mellitus are also reduced. Physical exercise should always be part of a treatment plan. The best type of physical exercise is daily walks for one hour and longer hikes as often as possible.

People who have to treat their diabetes with insulin (type 1 diabetes) should not exercise in the evening, in order to avoid hypoglycaemia at night. They should not inject insulin near strongly stressed muscle groups, where it will reach the blood more quickly (even if it is injected into the fat above) and may lead to hypoglycaemia. One to two bread units should be eaten before walks or physical exercise. It is advisable to carry raisins and glucose for emergencies while outdoors.

Movement must always be considered in treatment, either by reducing the insulin dose or by eating. This is taught in diabetes training, but requires significant personal experience.

Patients with type 1 diabetes can generally practice any sport. People with type 2 diabetes should practice dynamic sports such as hiking, swimming, dancing or cross-country skiing. They should avoid weight training while their blood pressure is still high.

Quitting smoking as part of the basic treatment for diabetes mellitus

Consuming tobacco increases insulin resistance[61,62]. Smoking is a danger for developing type 1 diabetes. It leads to the formation of numerous reactive oxygen species (ROS) and thus to strong oxidative stress as described above[63].

Oxidative stress is at the focus of the causes of the autoimmune reactions that destroy the beta cells of the pancreas and cause type 1 diabetes[64]. Smoking reduces the kidney function (glomerular filtration rate) in men with type 1 diabetes[65].

Many studies have proven smoking to be an important cause of type 2 diabetes. It doubles the risk of developing diabetes mellitus[66]. In a major Japanese study it was proven that this is independent of dosage. This means that it does not matter how many cigarettes are smoked every day. People aged 40 and up are particularly at risk[67].

Scientists explain the risk of diabetes by the oxidative stress caused by smoking, due to increase of the insulin resistance and because smoking clearly reduces the glucose transport in the skeletal muscles. In addition there is the direct toxic effect of the carbon monoxide and other substances in tobacco smoke on the islet cells of the pancreas[68]. It is particularly bad if one also drinks alcohol. Smoking increases the damage done even by small amounts of alcohol. We have already shown and explained why the risk of cardiovascular disease is strongly increased in diabetes. Smoking further potentiates this risk and increases damage to the kidneys.

Mortality risk due to damage to the cardiovascular system caused by smoking diminishes only slowly in the course of many years after quitting smoking. The longer a person has previously smoked[69, 70, 71] the slower it diminishes.

Quitting smoking is officially a basic measure to prevent and treat diabetes mellitus[72].

Diabetes and alcohol

It was long disputed among nutritionists whether there was any connection between alcohol consumption and diabetes mellitus. The frequency (prevalence) of diabetes mellitus tripled worldwide over the past three decades.

Epidemiological studies have shown that it is not genetic factors, but rather unhealthy diet, lack of movement, smoking and alcohol consumption that are at the focus of the causes for this increase. The strongest effect was found in Asia, and specifically in China and India, though western countries are affected nearly as much. The role of alcohol consumption is still under dispute. After drinking a small amount of alcohol, sensitivity of the cell membranes to insulin increases slightly. This must be considered when using insulin for treatment. The dose must be reduced by approx. 20 %. This initially led to the hypothesis that moderate alcohol consumption may even benefit the course of diabetes mellitus. However, occasional drinking to a certain intoxication clearly increases the diabetes risk in both men and women[73, 74]. After various epidemiological studies indicted a reduced risk of type 2 diabetes when occasionally drinking small amounts of alcohol[75, 76], large prospective studies that carefully cancelled out other risk factors showed that people who often drank small amounts of alcohol ("moderate and social drinkers") developed type 2 diabetes significantly more often than abstinent people[77, 78].

Looking at the question of alcohol in isolation, the wrong conclusions will be drawn.

The risk to people with diabetes mellitus is mostly in the secondary diseases. Most die of heart attack or stroke. All other risk factors for these disasters must also be considered. Regular small alcohol doses (i.e. a glass of red wine with dinner) will place considerable stress on the liver, the pancreas and the metabolism. Lifelong drinking of moderate alcohol amounts is an important partial cause for the metabolic syndrome, defined by the symptoms overweight, hypertension and fat metabolism disorder[79]. This is one of the most important risk factors for cardiovascular diseases, with the disastrous events of heart attack and stroke. The damage caused by regular small alcohol doses are described in detail in our Bircher-Benner manual no. 19 for patients with hypertension, cardiovascular disease and arteriosclerosis. Furthermore, moderate, regular consumption of alcohol will harm the kidneys, leading to more frequent and earlier development of diabetic nephropathy and renal insufficiency[80].

Coffee and diabetes mellitus

Considerable funds are required to perform a scientific study.

No other subjects bring as many contradictory results as alcohol and coffee. Usually the studies that show a positive effect on health appear first. Later they are relativised by newer studies that document harmful effects This was the case with coffee and its effect on people with diabetes mellitus.
A prospective study from 1986–1997 handed a questionnaire to 28,812 postmenopausal women who initially had neither diabetes, obesity or cardiovascular issues.

According to the answers of these women in the follow-up review with a second questionnaire 11 years later, those who said that they had drunk more decaffeinated coffee had developed type 2 diabetes mellitus a little less often than those who did not drink coffee at all[81]. The result was greatly noticed, in particular since it supported daily habits. Coffee supposedly not only protects against diabetes, but also against angina pectoris and heart attack, depression and even Alzheimer's dementia. More recently, these results have been brought into question by observation studies[82]. It has also been proven that drinking coffee increases the blood levels of cholesterol and apolipoprotein B in men, and that the risk of cardiovascular diseases such as heart attack and stroke is also increased[83, 84, 85]. This result is very important for people with type 2 diabetes, since their higher cardiovascular risk is at greatest risk for their health and lives.

Smoking and obesity cause genetic changes from genetic polymorphism. This means that the effects cause harmful genetic mutations over the course of people's lives. In 2015, the genetic changes caused by regular coffee consumption were examined. Genetic changes caused by coffee consumption were found to be similar to those caused by smoking and obesity. In animal tests, it was proven that coffee harms the intestinal flora, which increases insulin resistance[86]. Overall, there are not a great many scientific examinations of the effects of coffee consumption on the risk of diabetes, but the prevailing view today is one of harmful effects. Type 2 diabetes mellitus can be healed by diet as long as the islet cells of the pancreas have not been destroyed. Our many years of experience show that avoiding coffee and alcohol is a requirement for healing.

Treatment of type 2 diabetes according to the guidelines of the Deutsche Gesellschaft for Diabetes[87]

Because of dangerous secondary diseases, the medical school classifies type 2 diabetics as high-risk patients. The cornerstone of treatment for type 2 diabetes has been defined as weight reduction, increased exercise and improved diet. Other cardiovascular risk factors are also treated. Hypertension is treated with medication to be kept below 130/85 mm Hg if possible. Metabolic disorder is treated with statins, which are drugs that inhibit the cholesterol synthesis in the intestine and the liver. Urine is examined for albumin in order to recognise microalbuminuria as an early sign of kidney damage. Nevertheless, most patients who have to commence dialysis treatment due to renal failure today are people with type 2 diabetes.

Permanent reduction of the body weight is usually impossible, since this is mostly done by reducing calories. The biophysical knowledge on the quality of food energy and the decisive relevance of plant-based raw food for restoration of the metabolic disorder have not yet reached academic medicine.

Official recommendations for changing the diet and weight control	
Weight control	BMI < 25 Kg/m2 body surface Waist circumference: Women: < 80 cm Men: < 94 cm
Carbohydrates	50 %
Fat	35 %
Protein	15–20 %
Dietary fibres (fruit and vegetables): at least 30 g/day	
Limitation of the calorie intake to 2000 Kcal/day on average	
Sugar intake ≤ 50 g per day	
Fat intake: saturated fatty acids < 10 % of the total energy supply polyunsaturated fats < 10 % of the total energy supply hydrogenated plant-based fats should be avoided due to the transfer of fatty acids monounsaturated fatty acids are preferred (olive oil) limitation of the cholesterol intake to less than 300 mg per day	
Alcohol: Women ≤ 10 g pure alcohol per day Men ≤ 20 g pure alcohol per day	

Assessment of body weight
The body mass index (BMI) is used for this. It is calculated by taking the body weight in Kg and dividing by the squared body size:

Weight classification of adults based on BMI (according to WHO, as of 2008)[88]

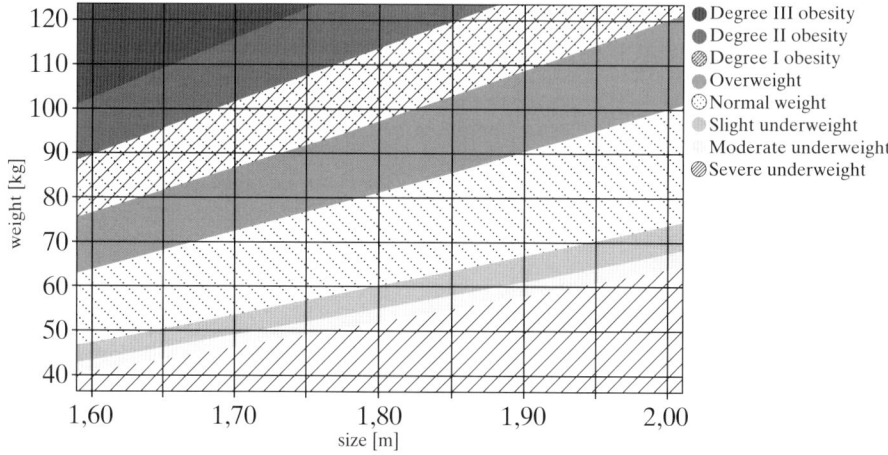

Weight classes depending on body mass and body size (according to adjacent BMI information)

Category	BMI (kg/m²)	Body weight
Severe underweight	< 16	
Moderate underweight	< 16,0 – < 17,0	Underweight
Slight underweight	< 17,0 – < 18,5	
Normal weight	< 18,5 – < 25,0	Normal weight
Pre-obesity	< 25,0 – < 30,0	Overweight
Degree I obesity	< 30,0 – < 35,0	
Degree II obesity	< 35,0 – < 40,0	Obesity
Degree III obesity	≥ 40	

The BMI is an excessive generalisation that does not consider gender, body structure or age. We recommend instead using our table on page 57 at the beginning of the diet section.

Diabetics who are treated with sulfonyl ureas, glinide or insulin must learn to plan their carbohydrate intake. They have to learn to handle bread units.
Drinking alcohol always creates a hypoglycaemia risk for them. Alcohol raises their triglyceride level. Therefore, even academic medicine recommends that patients with hypertriglyceridemia avoid alcohol entirely.

Tables for ideal weight

The ideal weight of adult men

Table 1a: Ideal weight of adult MEN
Ideal weight in kilograms, 25 years and older

Size cm	Light bone structure	Medium bone structure	Heavy bone structure
154	48.5 – 52.2	51.3 – 56.2	54.9 – 61.7
155	49.1 – 52.7	51.8 – 56.9	55.4 – 62.2
156	49.6 – 53.2	52.3 – 57.6	56.0 – 62.8
157	50.2 – 53.8	52.9 – 58.3	56.5 – 63.3
158	50.7 – 54.3	53.4 – 58.9	57.0 – 64.0
159	51.2 – 54.9	53.9 – 59.4	57.6 – 64.7
160	51.8 – 55.4	54.5 – 59.9	58.1 – 65.5
161	52.3 – 55.9	55.0 – 60.5	58.7 – 66.2
162	52.9 – 56.5	55.6 – 61.0	59.2 – 66.9
163	53.4 – 57.2	56.1 – 61.7	59.7 – 67.6
164	53.9 – 57.9	56.6 – 62.4	60.3 – 68.3
165	54.5 – 58.6	57.2 – 63.1	60.9 – 69.1
166	55.2 – 59.3	57.9 – 63.8	61.6 – 70.0
167	55.7 – 60.0	58.7 – 64.6	62.3 – 70.9
168	56.6 – 60.7	59.4 – 65.4	63.1 – 71.8
169	57.4 – 61.4	60.1 – 66.3	64.0 – 72.7
170	58.1 – 62.2	60.8 – 67.1	64.9 – 73.5
171	58.8 – 62.9	61.5 – 67.9	65.6 – 74.2
172	59.5 – 63.9	62.2 – 68.6	66.3 – 74.9
173	60.2 – 64.4	62.9 – 69.3	67.0 – 75.6
174	60.9 – 65.3	63.7 – 70.0	67.7 – 76.4
175	61.9 – 66.2	64.4 – 70.8	68.4 – 77.1
176	62.4 – 66.9	65.1 – 71.6	69.2 – 78.0
177	63.1 – 67.9	65.8 – 72.5	69.9 – 78.9
178	63.8 – 68.3	66.5 – 73.4	70.7 – 79.8
179	64.5 – 69.0	67.2 – 74.3	71.6 – 80.7
180	65.2 – 69.8	67.9 – 75.2	72.5 – 81.6
181	65.9 – 70.5	68.7 – 76.1	73.2 – 82.5

Size cm	Light bone structure	Medium bone structure	Heavy bone structure
182	66.6 – 71.2	69.4 – 77.0	73.9 – 83.4
183	69.4 – 72.0	70.1 – 77.9	74.7 – 84.2
184	68.1 – 72.9	70.8 – 78.8	75.6 – 85.1
185	68.8 – 73.8	71.5 – 79.7	76.5 – 86.0
186	69.5 – 74.5	72.4 – 80.6	77.4 – 86.9
187	70.2 – 75.2	73.3 – 81.5	78.3 – 87.8
188	70.9 – 75.9	74.2 – 82.4	79.1 – 88.7
189	71.6 – 76.6	75.1 – 83.3	79.8 – 89.6
190	72.4 – 77.3	76.0 – 84.1	80.5 – 90.5
191	73.1 – 78.1	76.9 – 85.0	81.2 – 91.4
192	73.8 – 78.8	77.8 – 85.9	82.0 – 92.3

Adjusted according to the *Statistical Bulletin*, vol. 40 (1959) of the Metropolitan Life Insurance Company
Ideal weight: weight with the longest life expectation

The ideal weight of adult women

Table 1b: Ideal weight of adults WOMEN
Ideal weight in kilograms, 25 years and older

Size cm	Light bone structure	Medium bone structure	Heavy bone structure
144	40.5 – 43.3	42.3 – 47.4	45.9 – 52.8
145	40.8 – 43.9	42.6 – 47.9	46.3 – 53.4
146	41.2 – 44.4	43.0 – 48.5	46.7 – 53.9
147	41.5 – 44.9	43.6 – 49.0	47.2 – 54.4
148	41.9 – 45.5	44.1 – 49.5	47.7 – 55.0
149	42.4 – 46.0	44.6 – 50.1	48.3 – 55.5
150	42.9 – 46.5	45.2 – 50.6	48.8 – 56.1
151	43.4 – 47.1	45.7 – 51.1	49.3 – 56.6
152	43.9 – 47.6	46.2 – 51.8	49.8 – 57.1
153	44.5 – 48.1	46.7 – 52.2	50.4 – 57.6
154	45.0 – 48.7	47.3 – 52.8	50.9 – 58.2
155	45.6 – 49.2	47.8 – 53.3	51.5 – 58.7
156	46.1 – 49.7	48.4 – 53.8	52.0 – 59.3
157	46.7 – 50.3	48.9 – 54.5	52.5 – 60.0
158	47.2 – 50.8	49.5 – 55.3	53.1 – 60.7
159	47.7 – 51.4	50.0 – 56.0	53.7 – 61.4

Size cm	Light bone structure	Medium bone structure	Heavy bone structure
160	48.3 – 51.9	50.5 – 56.7	54.4 – 62.2
161	48.8 – 52.4	51.1 – 57.4	55.2 – 62.9
162	49.3 – 53.1	51.8 – 58.3	55.8 – 63.6
163	49.9 – 53.8	52.5 – 59.2	56.6 – 64.3
164	50.5 – 54.5	53.2 – 60.0	57.3 – 65.0
165	51.2 – 55.3	53.9 – 60.7	58.0 – 65.7
166	51.9 – 56.0	54.6 – 61.4	58.7 – 66.4
167	52.6 – 56.7	55.3 – 62.1	59.4 – 67.1
168	53.3 – 57.4	56.0 – 62.8	60.1 – 67.8
169	54.0 – 58.1	56.8 – 63.6	60.8 – 68.6
170	54.8 – 58.8	57.5 – 64.3	61.6 – 69.3
171	55.5 – 59.5	58.2 – 65.0	62.3 – 70.0
172	56.2 – 60.4	58.9 – 65.7	63.0 – 70.8
173	56.9 – 61.3	59.6 – 66.3	63.7 – 71.7
174	57.6 – 62.1	60.3 – 67.1	64.4 – 72.6
175	58.3 – 62.9	61.0 – 67.8	65.1 – 73.5
176	59.0 – 63.6	61.8 – 68.6	65.8 – 74.4
177	59.8 – 64.3	62.5 – 69.3	66.6 – 75.3
178	60.5 – 65.0	63.2 – 70.0	67.3 – 76.2
179	61.2 – 65.7	63.9 – 70.7	68.0 – 77.1
180	61.9 – 66.4	64.6 – 71.4	68.7 – 78.0
181	62.6 – 67.1	65.3 – 72.1	69.4 – 78.9

Adjusted according to the *Statistical Bulletin*, vol. 40 (1959) of the Metropolitan Life Insurance Company
Ideal weight: weight with the longest life expectation

The strictly thermal food energy in kilocalories:

The energy content of the three food types and alcohol	
Fats	9 Kcal pro per gram
Carbohydrates	4 Kcal pro per gram
Proteins	4 Kcal pro per gram
Alcohol	7 Kcal pro per gram

This information is not strictly correct. The figures have been rounded down to simplify calculation.

The problem of food energy

Officially recognised dietary recommendations are based on understanding food energy in the form of pure heat energy (calories), and thus the first law of thermodynamics, phrased in 1842 by German doctor Julius Robert Mayer. It was the basis for formulation of the law on preservation of energy by Hermann von Helmholz in 1847, and states that calorific energy is never lost in a closed system during mechanical or chemical processes (i.e. it is always preserved). In

1865, German physicist Rudolf Clausius found the contradiction between the first law of thermodynamics and reality, and formulated the second law of thermodynamics, stating that the thermal energy in a closed system may not be lost, but that physical disorder happens in any spontaneously occurring chemical or mechanical processes. He called this entropy and thus proved that perpetuum mobile (a motor running without energy supply) is impossible.

Clausius marked the beginning of a new understanding of the quality of energies. These findings were included in the sciences of chemistry and physics, but surprisingly never in medicine and nutrition. Maximilian Bircher-Benner corrected this in his teachings on food, published in Berlin in 1905. He applied the second law of thermodynamics to food energy[89, 90]. Living foods made of plants that have photosynthesis were assigned the highest available food energy. (See "Two kinds of food energy" below).

Bircher-Benner's understanding of food energy by its qualitative value has been confirmed in all respects by recent research in biophysics, biophoton research and molecular biology[91, 92, 93, 94, 95, 96, 97].

The biophysical quality and order of foods forms the basis of the nutritional science underlying this book. The surprising deficit of the current medical paradigm concerning these findings is the reason why permanent healing of obesity and type 2 diabetes is usually impossible according to widespread methodology. Results are quite different when the Bircher-Benner diet described in this book is adhered to.
The widespread methodology has tragic consequences, since today patients are usually treated with medicines. These cannot heal type 2 diabetes, unfortunately, and at best slightly delay the secondary diseases. Many dangerous side effects of medicines compound the basic issue of diabetes.

Diabetes medicines (antidiabetics), effect and side effects

There are medicines that force the beta cells in the pancreas to produce more insulin (insulinotropic antidiabetics). They pose a risk of hypoglycaemias as soon as food intake is decreased even slightly. In type 2 diabetes, the islet cells are already overloaded, since they have to produce more insulin than usual because of insulin resistance. They will be exhausted over time. This can be seen when the previously raised insulin level drops below the standard.

Non-insulinotropic antidiabetics

These drugs do not stimulate insulin release, so that the risk of hypoglycaemia is low and the islet cells are exhausted less quickly. The following type of antidiabetic is therefore preferred:

Metformin
In type 2 diabetes mellitus, glucose cannot reach the liver cells because of insulin resistance. Consequently the liver cells register a lack of glucose, which causes them to produce excess glucose and discharge it into the blood.

Metformin inhibits the formation of new glucose (gluconeogenesis) in the liver Unpleasant side effects include nausea, pain in the upper abdomen and rarely over-acidification of the body with lactic acid (lactic acidosis). Because of these side effects, metformin is best taken at the end of a meal.

Metformin is used in case of insulin resistance. It must not be taken if creatinine values are greater than 106 umol/l, which would indicate kidney damage (nephropathy). Other counterindications include liver damage, inflammation of the pancreas (pancreatitis), alcoholism, oxygen deficit in the blood (hypoxia), pregnancy and lactation, and (during weight reduction) diets of less than 1000 Kcal.

Alpha glucosidase inhibitors (Acarbose [Glucobay®], Miglitol [Diastabol®])
These drugs inhibit the alpha-glucosidase enzyme in the intestine. It is necessary for breaking down polysaccharides into single sugar molecules (monosaccharides). This slows sugar resorption in the intestine, so that the blood sugar increase is slower after a meal and will be reduced in general. They are used if high glucose values are measured after meals.
They must be taken with the first bite of the meal so that they reach the intestine with the meal.
They cause flatulence and diarrhoea as side effects.

Alpha-glucosidase inhibitors are prohibited for patients younger than 18 or in cases of chronic intestinal diseases, progressed nephropathy with partial kidney failure (renal insufficiency), pregnancy and lactation.
Many patients do not take these medicines for long, since they have unpleasant side effects. Their effect is also questionable (Stop-NIDDM study)[98, 99].

Glitazone (Pioglitazone [Actos®], Rosiglitazone [Avandia®])
These drugs increase sensitivity of all cells to insulin by amplifying the GLUT1 and

GLUT4 transport systems for glucose in the cell membranes. This is specifically the case in the muscle cells.
They are also used to reduce insulin resistance.
For overweight patients, they are combined with metformin (e.g. Avandamet®, Competact®).
They can have relevant and dangerous adverse effects, such as weight increase, oedemas (water deposits in the tissue), liver damage and increased brittle bones in women.
Counterindications: pregnancy, lactation, heart failure and nephropathy with severe renal insufficiency, and function impairment of the liver (raised liver enzyme values).
For these two drugs (without the addition of metformin), studies are available that document positive effects in which they are superior to other antidiabetics, including metformin. They supposedly inhibit inflammation (reduction of the C-reactive protein CRP and the leukocyte number) and inhibit fattening of the liver. On the other hand, the hormone adiponectin is increased, which causes excess storage of fat cells and fat in the body. This includes fat cells that are already overly filled, which increases body weight[100, 101, 102].

Insulinotropic antidiabetics

These drugs are used in patients with normal weight who have developed insulin-resistance due to poor nutrition, and therefore have an increased insulin demand. They suffer from a relative insulin deficit as compared to their increased demand. They are unsuitable for overweight people since they cause body weight to increase.

Sulfonyl-urea derivatives ([Clibenclamid], Glimepiride [Amaryl®] etc.)
These drugs force the beta cells of the pancreas, which are already overloaded, to produce even more insulin.

The adverse effects are considerable. There is a risk of dangerous hypoglycaemia as soon as food intake is reduced slightly. Sulfonylureas with long-term effects are even more dangerous. These drugs cause an average weight increase of 4.8 kg over three years. This is absolutely undesirable and increases the risk of the dangerous secondary diseases of diabetes mellitus. The effect also reduces gradually over time.

Counterindications: pregnancy and lactation, larger surgeries, larger metabolic disorders, renal insufficiency (raised creatinine), liver insufficiency (raised liver enzymes) and allergic reactions to sulfonyl urea derivatives or probenecid (a drug prescribed against gout to reduce the urea level). This is a cross-sensitivity.

Glinides (Nateglinid [Starlix®], Repaglinide [NovoNorm®] etc.)
Glinides stimulate insulin from the beta cells of the pancreas more quickly than sulfonylurea derivatives.
The predominant side effect is a risk of hypoglycaemia, even if this is slightly less than in sulfonylurea derivatives. Weight gain is considerably less.
Counterindications: pregnancy and lactation, liver or renal insufficiency, allergies to these substances. Repaglinide must not be taken with Gemfibrozil (Gevilon®).

On insulin therapy in type 2 diabetes

Heart attack or stroke used to be the absolute indication for starting insulin therapy. Today strict measures to generally improve metabolism are preferred, on the basis of the results of a widespread study (DIGAMI-2 study[103]).

Hypoglycaemia

This indicates an insufficient blood sugar level (< 2.77 mmol/l or 50 mg/dl). When it is severe enough for a patient to faint, it is also called "sugar shock".

The point at which symptoms are felt differs from person to person. In addition to "asymptomatic hypoglycaemia", "symptomatic hypoglycaemia" has two degrees of severity:

a) it is still possible to recover from hypoglycaemia unassisted;
b) outside help is required.

Signs of hypoglycaemia include weakness, cold sweat, drowsiness and even unconsciousness. Sustained severe hypoglycaemia with unconsciousness can be life-threatening without immediate treatment. Hypoglycaemia in diabetes results from excessive insulin doses as compared to food intake, from overdosing on the above insulinotropic antidiabetics if physical exercise has not been sufficiently considered, or from alcohol.

In Great Britain, estimates suggest that more than 5,000 diabetics treated with sulfonylureas suffer severe hypoglycaemia ever year and must be rescued by emergency services[104].

After many years of insulin therapy for type 1 diabetes, hypoglycaemia increases in frequency, since the pancreas is less able to produce the glucagon antagonist. Patients who keep their glucose levels very low to prevent the secondary diseases also show an increased level of the adrenalin antagonist, which prevents them from noticing the hypoglycaemia symptoms until they suddenly fall unconscious.

Treatment of hypoglycaemia

As soon as the first symptoms are noticed, the patient should drink a little apple juice, eat a banana or, if he happens away from the home, have some glucose or eat some raisins, which should always be kept at hand.
The patient should then measure the blood sugar at once and find the possible cause.
In severe cases in which the patient cannot help himself anymore, glucose is placed in the mouth. The emergency doctor will inject glucagon intramuscular at once and place an IV for quick glucose supply. In such situations, hospitalisation is always necessary for monitoring and precise treatment.

Order therapy for diabetes mellitus

Basics to understand the causes and nutritional treatment of diabetes mellitus

Two kinds of food energy

Physicists have identified two types of energy: orderly and chaotic. Orderly energy saves information. Chaotic energy cannot save anything. Heat energy (calories) is chaotic energy. Sunlight is the most highly ordered form of energy. Its complex information content is like a large symphony. Listening to a symphony does not produce heat, but it provides information; it is a highly orderly sound structure that triggers precise sensations and feelings. With its complex oscillations, sunlight conveys and orders the genetically specified information that is needed for growth, differentiation and regeneration of all life on earth.

One green leaf contains about a hundred thousand chlorophyll funnels. At the base of each funnel, there are two chlorophyll α-molecules each. The funnel reflects the incoming light into the base, where the two chlorophyll α-molecules enter a maximum resonance, synchronised with the oscillations of the solar radiation. Physicists call this "coherence", in which the waves of sunlight become standing light waves called photons. Their energy, and therefore the information and resonance from sunlight, flows through the entire plant body, all the way down to the roots. Only a little of it is emitted as UV light, and it is invisible to the human eye.

All living cells store UV light in their molecules, particularly in the ring-shaped (aromatic) molecules. The double helix of the genetic material in the cell cores of deoxyribonucleic acid (DNA) stores the most light by far. The double helix can coil to the right or left and can form protrusions shaped like clover leaves, radiating specific UV light spectrums. The wound double helix of the DNA serves as a cavity resonator for the rhythmic amplification of UV light in vital cells. Amplification takes place rhythmically according to the laser principle. For a laser to take up work, it must receive a certain basic amount of energy. Physicists call this minimally necessary energy the "laser threshold". In their experiments, researchers of the international academy for biophoton research measured the laser threshold in plant-based cell tissues[93].

Just like plants, human and animal cells are formations of light while they are alive. This is the difference between life and death. They also store light as UV light[90] in their genetic material deoxyribonucleic acid (DNA). We lack the ability to photosynthesise, however, and direct application of sunlight to the skin is far from enough to keep our light storage above the laser threshold.
Plant cells store the photons from sunlight in incredible amounts. It could be shown that the ultra-weak cell radiation[91] is nothing but a radiation leakage, a tiny leak of UV light through the cell membrane. Measurements showed that laser amplification of the light is 10^4 times stronger in the DNA than that provided by the best technical laser devices. The

inside of cells therefore represents an incredible light space.

Our photon storage must be fed daily with a sufficient amount of vital photon-containing foods, i.e. fresh vegetable foods.

The transmission of the information of the vital foods from photosynthesis to our organism takes place by information transfer (or coherence), just as during photosynthesis. This means that our own sensation of life, life energy and life information is renewed and reordered again and again in the roughly 50 trillion cells of our body by entering into a shared resonance with the oscillation patterns and complex information of sunlight when the photons are transferred.

Energy inside the cell is very different from that of a non-living nature. Biophysicists call the inside of the cell a dissipative system, which is an ordered structure found in systems that are formed far from the thermodynamic equilibrium. Russian-Belgian researcher Ilya Prigogine received a Nobel prize for his work on this.

Intense photon storage removes the energy inside the cell so far from the thermodynamic balance that the second law of thermodynamics no longer applies. Thus the principle of chaos, which is valid outside all living things, becomes an ordering principle. Prigogine called this the coherence principle[96].

When living foods are missing from our nutrition, the photon content in our cells declines. The light content falls until it drops below the laser threshold. The cells partially revert from the principle of order (Prigogine's coherence principle) to the chaos principle of thermodynamics, and then they degenerate.

We consider disease a loss of order, a loss of ordered information. The programme of life enters into disorder, and the lack of living nutrition makes reordering impossible. Many experiments, conducted at the University of Novosibirsk and elsewhere[105, 106, 107] show that the complex processes of biochemistry in our cells are controlled by information. If there is a lack of living nutrition, this information provided by the genes in the DNA will no longer be continually renewed and ordered. Thus, the complex biochemical processes of our cells will be thrown into disarray. This is why living raw plant food is important for its energy: it renews and strengthens the ordering resonance in the biological system.

The basic regulation system of the soft connective tissue

All cells of the body's organs are embedded in the intercellular substance of the soft connective tissue that runs through all organs and structures. It consists of a dense molecular network (matrix) of sugar-protein molecules called proteoglycans, and is soaked with a rich liquid (interstitial fluid). The soft connective tissue contains spindle-shaped cells that form the network of the intercellular substance and continually adjust it as needed. The blood capillaries run through this intercellular substance with their network, including the nerve endings of the vegetative nervous system. Outside the brain and spinal cord, the capillaries deliberately leak, allowing the nutrients and hormones from the blood to leave the capillaries and enter the intercellular substances. They reach the cells through the molecular network, serving as a molecular sieve. At the same time, it is our system for conducting and storing biological information – the information in our living organism. There is no direct contact between the blood capillaries and the cells in our bodies, where they penetrate the intercellular substance and loop to the discharging veins there. The intercellular substance is drained by the complex system of lymph vessels and cleansed in the lymph nodes. It is then returned to the venous blood as purified lymph through the large lymph vessels. The nerves have blind ends in the intercellular substance.

All information from the nervous system to the cells, and from the cells to the nervous system, is routed through the proteoglycans molecular network. As a result, every piece of information is disseminated through the entire body: The system always reacts as a whole (e.g. acupuncture makes use of this). This complex system is our "basic regulation system"[108]. All cells in our bodies are supplied with biological information, hormones, nutrients and oxygen through the intercellular substance and the network of proteoglycan molecules.

The meaning of food economy[109]

Food economy means that the composition of food must correspond exactly to our biological needs, so that neither too much nor too little is supplied. The body needs very little food, but its composition must be adapted to the biologically given need as precisely as possible. Our biological system cannot cope with an excess of senselessly supplied nutrients. Such excess produces all the "civilisation diseases" that fill our hospitals and medical practices.

Food economy and food energy are decisive in keeping the complex intercellular substance and our basic regulation system healthy, both in the body and in the central nervous system beyond the blood-brain barrier.
Senselessly and excessively supplied nutrients and toxins from a diseased, overloaded, overacidified metabolism and a sick environment in the stomach and intestines cannot be managed or excreted. They remain in the complex system of the intercellular substance as degenerative metabolic slags. There they gradually hinder the vital exchange of substances, gases, and the storage and flow of biological information. The intercellular substance (also called matrix) is where the entire morbidity of "civilised man" – the civilised diseases – develop.

The system of basic regulation also includes the environment inside the intestine, with its immense ecosystem of intestinal flora. We have seen that autoimmune processes from an ill milieu in the intestine and a degenerated intestinal flora are supported because the immune cells can only acquire defective immune competence under such conditions to distinguish properly between external and internal – between useful and harmful. A diseased environment in the intestine is a huge interference field that strongly impairs the basic regulation of the whole organism. Rot toxins formed by anaerobic bacteria reach the liver through the oral vein system, together with the uselessly supplied nutrients, and overload it massively. They slag down its intercellular substance until the innermost liver cells of the liver lobules die and are replaced by fat cells. This is how fatty liver develops. Anything that it cannot detoxify and make water-soluble goes back into the intestine via the bile ducts. From there it is returned to the liver over and over, to try to detoxify the material. Thus rot toxins and excessive nutrients continue to circulate between the intestine and the liver (enterohepatic circulation), and they overload it. Haemorrhoids are caused by overloading of the veins of the rectum, as they are connected to the portal vein system.

In addition, generally widespread malnutrition, with its excess of protein, fat and sugars in the metabolism, produces huge amounts of organic acids, strongly oxidising ketonic acids and other ROS (reactive oxygen species).

These massively overtax our antioxidative systems. (See the chapter on oxidative stress and its consequences). Oxidation means degeneration. Proteins modified by oxidation are oxidised. They become insoluble and are deposited in the intercellular substance of the entire body as amyloids. They oxidise cholesterol, which is protected by unsaturated fatty acids inside the LDL molecule on its transport to the cell membranes in the blood. Oxidation makes it insoluble. It accumulates in the arteries and heart in places of rapid blood flow (fatty streaks). Today this happens at a young age, at the onset of arteriosclerosis. ROS oxidise proteins, making them insoluble and causing them to deposit in the network structure of the intercellular substance as amyloids. The deposition of such β-Amyloid and TAU proteins in the intercellular substance of the brain causes Alzheimer's disease; in the arteries it causes arteriosclerosis, heart attack and stroke; in the veins it causes varicose veins; in the synovial layer of the joints it causes arthritis; in the coils of the renal capillaries (glomeruli) it causes nephrosis, all the way to diabetic kidney failure; in the finer connective-tissue structure of the bones and cartilages it causes osteoporosis and arthrosis; in the thyroid it causes Hashimoto or Badsedow's inflammation; and in the eyes it causes glaucoma and cataract, or degeneration of the retina (macular degeneration). If the regulatory capacity of the biological system collapses, cancer develops because the immune system is no longer able to recognise and eliminate the cancer cells that develop every day.

The immune system recognises all degenerative changes of molecules as foreign so that autoimmune reactions increase, in a failed attempt of the immune system to destroy the seemingly foreign substances, and so that the degenerative phenomena are additionally accelerated by autoimmune inflammations, as we have seen in type 1 diabetes.

The integral law of nutrition[110]

The composition of the ingredients of the plant foods stipulated by nature corresponds most precisely to the biologically specified requirements. It must be noted that different parts of the plants – the flowers, fruits, kernels, nuts, leaves, stems and roots – contain different substances. Toxic fractions must be avoided. If this is taken into account, the demand for food economy is most likely to be met if the plant is regarded as integral, and if all parts of its diet are taken into account.

Vibrancy of food

As we have seen, a high energy potential – a high proportion of living food from plants that are capable of photosynthesis – is of great importance in the fight against all degenerative diseases. This is due to their regenerative effect from a high content of stored photons, i.e. the complex information from sunlight that regulates the biological system. In diabetes mellitus, a high share of living, plant-based fresh foods (raw food) of at least 70 %, and at the beginning of every meal, is decisive for healing. Vitamin B_{12}, which does not occur in plants, must be supplemented. As long as insulin-resistance persists, a strict raw food diet consisting of living plant-based foods, plant milk and nuts over several months is most effective. It also contains the plant substances with a pharmacological effect, the so-called secondary plant substances (phytochemicals) in their purest form.

Secondary plant substances (phytochemicals) with an antidiabetic effect

As already described, diabetes mellitus requires a choice of food with a low glycaemic index (GI). These are foods with high fibre content. They release their sugars more slowly into the blood, keeping the blood sugar level increase as flat as possible. The GI compares the blood sugar increase of a food to that provided by the same amount of carbohydrates in the form of pure glucose.

For example, fresh grain, peanuts and lentils, as well as fructose that enters the cells without insulin, all have a GI of 40 %. Rye grain, yoghurt and milk, peas, dried beans, apples, spaghetti, orange juice and oranges have a GI of 60 %. Wholemeal bread, natural rice, oat flakes, rye bread, kitchen sugar have a GI of 80 %. Crispbread, potatoes and potato mash, white bread, maize and cornflakes have a GI of 95 %. The GI of glucose or maltose is 100 %.

In addition to the dietary fibres, other food components influence the conversion of plant starch into glucose. This includes the polyphenols of the outer layers of fruits and vegetables, the partially heat-labile lectins of legumes, the phytic acid from outer layers of whole grains, legumes and oil seeds, and the protease inhibitors of fresh soy beans, mung beans, garden peas, peanuts, potatoes, whole rice, corn, oats and whole wheat. The glycaemic index (i.e. the glucose stress on the metabolism) can be strongly influenced by this so that the foods are broken down as little as possible by food processing, and eaten in as natural a condition as possible (i.e. without being pureed or mixed). Wheat and legumes contain amylase inhibitors. These are substances that inhibit the activity of the enzyme amylase, so that the starch will be broken down into sugar less quickly. They are found in the seeds of grains and legumes. Amylase inhibitors are heat-sensitive except for wheat, where they can still be found in baked wholemeal bread. Legumes also contain tannins which slow down starch digestion and are still 50 % effective after cooking. It has been scientifically recognised that vegetable nutrition especially with wholemeal and legumes reduces the blood sugar curve. The diet also requires consideration of 1) all secondary plant substances (phytochemicals) that contribute to the prevention of the secondary diseases of diabetes mellitus; 2) plant substances with strong antioxidative effects which reduce blood pressure and cholesterol; and 3) immunomodulating substances. We refer here to the Bircher-Benner manual no. 4 on fresh juices, raw vegetable and fruit dishes. That book is a great help for raw food therapy for diabetes mellitus.

The effects of diet and medication are revealed only if the body cells have been made receptive in advance by "nutritive stimulus". In addition to the diet, this is triggered by the influence of light, air, water and physical activity. Mental attitude also has a great influence on the healing process. Adjusting the dosage of this "stimulus" can make a great contribution to healing. One must be aware that weak stimuli increase vitality, medium stimuli promote it, while strong stimuli inhibit vitality, here as elsewhere.

The mineral metabolism in diabetes mellitus

The metabolic disorder of diabetes also affects minerals and trace elements. This was long underestimated. Disorders in the electrolyte balance, calcium, phosphate and potassium are formed when the blood sugar level is high. Ketoacidosis (overacidification with keto bodies), for which type 1 diabetics are at risk, causes potassium to be lost. This is also the case in type 2 diabetics when it is treated badly. As long as type 2 diabetes is not healed or well managed, diabetics are particularly at risk for zinc and magnesium deficits. However, these minerals may only be supplemented if there is a proven deficiency. There is scientific evidence that a magnesium deficiency in the diet has a negative effect on blood sugar control.

Green leaves contain magnesium in the chlorophyll molecule in biologically optimal availability. Therefore our diet is ideal for this correction. By contrast, there is no scientific evidence that medicinal magnesium supplementation is effective. The osteoporosis risk is increased in type 2 diabetes[111].

The blood levels of various micronutrients in diabetes are often altered in the long term. However, it cannot be concluded from this that there is excess or deficiency, since these blood levels reflect the profound regulatory disorder in this disease. Diabetes mellitus shows autoantibodies against the zinc transporter ZnT8. These can be found in 98 % of type 2 patients at the very onset, and therefore can be used for early diagnosis[112]. Type 2 diabetes usually comes with a zinc deficit, even though only about 10 % of patients show these antibodies, with increased copper and iron levels (ferritin)[113]. Zinc deficiency worsens every year[114,115]. Certain rheumatism medicines, antibiotics and tuberculosis medicines, as well as other medicines and alcohol, intensify the zinc deficiency. Zinc-rich foods include wholemeal (2.4 mg/100 g), wholemeal oat flakes (14 mg/100 g), nuts (2.4 mg/100 g) and legumes (2–9 mg/100 g), while white flour and coloured sugar contain no zinc or other trace elements. This illustrates the great importance of whole foods. It has been shown that the correction of zinc levels contributes to better blood sugar control. There is often a deficiency of the trace element chromium[116]. However, clinical studies evaluating the effect of chromium supplementation on blood glucose control have shown contradictory results. Even though a large amount of experimental data suggests an important role of chromium in the insulin and glucose metabolism, there is no consistent clinical evidence that chrome preparations would be effective in diabetes. Thus they cannot be recommended at the present time. It is not yet certain whether vanadium is an essential (necessary) trace element. The administration of vanadyl sulphate showed a positive effect on blood sugar control in type 2 diabetes in some studies. However, we have no data yet about compatibility after long-term use. It therefore cannot be recommended at this time. Taking iron, copper and selenium without previous examination and careful monitoring of the blood levels may have a negative effect in diabetes mellitus, and should be avoided.

Medicinal herbs for treating diabetes

Folk medicine has always known medicinal herbs for diabetes mellitus. They are chosen based on centuries-old recommendations. The ingredients and their mode of action have usually been insufficiently researched. Although they cannot cure diabetes on their own, they can be used to support a diet.

Various plants contain glycokines with a weak insulin effect. They are found in bean shell extract, available as for example Phaseolan fluidum Tosse. Galega (Galea officinalis) contains the glycokine galegin, a guanidine compound with a mild insulin effect. It is used as galega tea. If the patient is underweight, it helps to maintain body weight. Galega tea shows some effect against acidosis in severe cases, and is also supposed to promote the incorporation of glycogen in the liver. It tastes a little strange. Silubin® capsules contain corresponding guanine compounds (biguanides). Their effect is deemed proven. The biguanides speed up absorption of glucose in the cells after a meal. This saves insulin and converts less glucose to fat. As a result, less fatty tissue is formed. Biguanides can be used as a dietary supplement against obesity.

Two other medicinal plants from India contain valuable glycokines. One is the popular Indian kidney tea "Koemis Koetjing" from Folia Orthosiphonis staminei. Besides essential oils, it contains fat-soluble flavones and 3 % potassium salts. In addition to the insulin-saving effect, it is deemed a diuretic, anti-inflammatory and cramp-reliever. Therefore it is particularly useful for diabetic nephropathy.

In India the fruits of the Syzygium jambolana tree, in the form of tea, are also used as glycokines against diabetes. Bitter melon (Momordica charantia), also called bitter cucumber or bitter gourd, contains several antidiabetic substances, such as charantin and p-insulin with an insulin-like effect. The tea should be prepared so that it tastes pleasant instead of bitter. No more than one litre of it is permitted per day, since an overdose can cause gastrointestinal problems. It is not recommended for pregnant women. Golden-yellow cinquefoil *(Potentilla aurea)*, the seeds and leaves of galega *(Galega officinalis)*, thorny burnet *(Poterium spinosum)* and copalchi *(Coutarea latifolia)* are also recommended to treat diabetes.

Other substances with a glycokine-like effect can be found in the extract of raw artichokes, blueberry leaf tea, chicory root, onion, stinging nettle, oats, oranges and lemons, celery, cabbage and lettuce, Jerusalem artichokes, sunflowers etc., which should be taken into account in the diet.

The meaning of movement

Exercise reduces the need for insulin. This must be considered in insulin treatment. Daily hiking clearly and permanently reduces the blood sugar level and lowers the HbA1c level. This is particularly important for the prevention of secondary[117] diseases[118, 119, 120]. Different types of movement make sense. Moderate exercise is more effective than weight training and competitive sports. A daily hike of at least one hour is always part of the therapy plan. Moderate walking up a modest incline in light clothing is ideal. For holidays and spa stays, it is important to pay attention to the severity of climate stimuli. Low mountain ranges (i.e. between 600 and 800 m above sea level) and the Baltic Sea offer medium-strong stimuli. They are particularly suitable for people who suffer from heart conditions. The high mountains (i.e. greater than 1000 m above sea level) and the North Sea are strongly stimulating climates. While unsuitable for patients with heart disease, they are ideal for allergies, asthma and other lung ailments, for weakened people, and where no symptoms exist yet.

General directives for order therapy for diabetes

The cornerstones of the therapy are:
- the diet described in this book;
- physical training;
- order of life;
- physical and mental hygiene;
- medicines, if they cannot be avoided.

Regarding the diet

Since the discovery of insulin in 1921, it has been believed that this magic formula could help patients avoid all dietary restrictions. Dietetics became the stepchild of diabetes treatment, so much so that to this day medical studies only provide rudimentary knowledge of dietetics. For about 50 years, however, we have been aware that diet must be the basis for all further diabetes treatments. After the emergence of insulin, diabetic treatment was attempted according to the principle of "eat little, avoid sugar and replace fat with protein" to stay alive for as long as possible.

In 1900, it had become clear that the diabetic needs the carbohydrates which are lost in this diet. Oat days were introduced, with which some diabetics who were believed lost could recover for a while. This was the first step towards realising that carbohydrates in their natural form had a different effect from denatured sugars and flours, and that the latter did harm. Then it was gradually recognised that the then-recommended excess of protein, meat and eggs promoted longer-term damage and produced a flood of uric acid (gout), which further damaged the islet cell apparatus. It was found that the amino acids from the excessively supposed protein had to be deaminated and converted into glucose on a complicated path that put a great strain on the metabolism. This overload on the metabolism caused the disease to worsen (e.g. 1 g glucose is made up of 3 g protein, or 4.86 g fat). In addition, this uneconomic conversion consumes considerable amounts of vitamin B_1 and B_6, which diabetics usually lack severely. The conversion of fat and protein into carbohydrates is enormously complex and takes considerable energy from the organism. The metabolism resembles a smouldering fire instead of a bright, clear flame. Not only is insulin missing, but so is the "coal" provided by carbohydrates.

When a diabetic body with low insulin levels was given few carbohydrates, replaced by protein and fat (as used to be common), patients also developed potassium, vitamin and mineral substance deficits and massive over-acidification from metabolic slags. It was finally discovered that over-feeding with fat without sufficient high-quality carbohydrates that are broken down slowly will poison the body with keto bodies, which may even lead to diabetic coma.

A diabetic who takes sleeping pills, painkillers and stimulants, increases his excessive thirst with salty food and tries to quench it with alcoholic drinks will harm his liver, kidneys, pancreas, vascular system and heart, which are already at the limits of their capacities. The patient then falls into the drama of secondary diseases caused by early degeneration. The limits of danger from degenerative "civilisation diseases" of the heart, brain, liver, kidneys and joints may be much narrower with diabetes mellitus. More than any other metabolic disease, diabetes requires the return to simple, high-energy nutrition that 1) is biologically economical, natural and low in amount; 2) lets the metabolism run economically, without toxins and harmoniously; and 3) prevents the deposit of metabolic slags in the soft connective tissue. These conditions are ideally met by the fresh plant-based diet described in this book.

As already described, fruits and vegetables contain substances that stimulate insulin from the insulin-forming beta cells of the pancreas, thereby countering the ketonic acid flood and metabolic disorder (antiketogenic effect). Fructose can be used for sweetening in small quantities. In contrast to glucose, fructose can enter the cells without insulin. Larger amounts must be avoided, since a high fructose level in the blood will damage the inner layer of the vessels more than glucose due to the phenomenon of glycation as described above. Sweetness in fruits, and partly also in honey, comes from fructose (also called laevulose). Sorbitol was originally found in the rowan tree. Like fructose, this natural sugar enters cells without insulin. Artificially produced, it is added to many diabetic foods today. Sorbitol has about one-third the sweetness of kitchen sugar. It is found in many fruits, especially in pome fruits (e.g. pears, plums, apples, apricots and peaches). In contrast, berries, citrus fruits, pineapples and grapes contain very little or no sorbitol[121]. At higher dosages, sorbitol also causes non-enzymatic glycation and damage to the inner layer of the blood vessels[122, 123]. It therefore must be used very sparingly, as it is also contained in fruits at low levels only. These sugar types are particularly suitable for the prevention of an acid coma that can easily occur in youthful and lean type 1 diabetics. A liver damaged by diabetes will most easily take up these sugar types without insulin to form its protection substance glycogen from them. This reduces the risk of rising cholesterol levels.

At present, academic medicine is focusing on improving drug therapy, and is trying to approximate the diet as closely as possible to the general malnutrition in order to restrict the patients in their diet as little as possible. Prevention and treatment of the causes is neglected. The result is a worldwide, steady increase in the number of diabetes cases and its complications. This is of little use to mankind. The new, healthy way of eating is easy to get used to in just a few weeks. Patients will gladly continue it, since they will be rewarded with a new, previously unknown sense of well-being and entirely new capacities, as well as by a decrease of familiar fatigue, headaches and other pains, improved sleep and mood, and a new resistance to colds and other infections.

Basic research and clinical and epidemiological work have laid the foundation for change of attitude, for tracking the causes in childhood, and for a completely different, new diet, as described in our manuals. The diet should consist of three meals for healthy people. Diabetics, however, need smaller main meals and small interim meals to balance out their blood sugar level and insulin demand. Our hormone levels are determined by the position of the sun and the diurnal cycle. They are highest at noon. That is why it is biologically specified that the main meal be consumed at noon, with a light, frugal side meal in the morning and evening each and two to three additional small snacks for the diabetic. Every meal must begin with fruit because of its high content of flavonoids that protect against cancer, and that are effective only for about four hours. Fruit is rich in enzymes, making it easy to digest. It does not remain in the stomach, especially if taken with something to drink. Nuts and almonds can be enjoyed with the fruit. The fruit reaches the duodenum directly and maintains a healthy intestinal flora throughout the intestine. Salad and raw vegetables should follow for lunch, finely and tastefully prepared and arranged. Since this food remains in the stomach for a longer time, one should not drink any more in order to not dilute the acid and digestive enzymes in the stomach. Only cold-pressed vegetable oils (e.g. sesame, sunflower, rapeseed, thistle, olive) should be used for salad dressings. Always add one-third linseed oil to ensure the content of omega-3 fatty acids. Olive oil contains predominantly monounsaturated fatty acids. In contrast to all polyunsaturated vegetable oils, olive oil may be heated (up to 170+°C) and served with warm food. Cooked food is not necessary, but it is pleasant for the main meal, particularly in winter. In order to stay healthy, cooked food should be the second choice after raw food and make up no more than 30 % of the meal. One or two vegetables and some wholemeal rice, potatoes, corn, millet, quinoa or barley in wholemeal quality, prepared in a pressure cooker or steamer, are best. Salt must be used sparingly, especially with high blood pressure. Rock salt must be given priority over sea salt, because of water pollution. It is possible to cook very tasty meals with little salt and instead achieve a rich, fragrant taste with onions, garlic and any number of herbs. This is easy to learn. Please refer to our Bircher-Benner manual no. 9 on enjoying food without table salt, with proven recipes from the famous Bircher-Benner Medical Centre. For breakfast, Bircher müesli according to the original recipe in this book is particularly suitable, with almond puree and freshly prepared almond or sesame milk. This fruit dish contains fructose from the fruit. It requires little insulin and will keep the eater satiated until lunch. All irritants, such as caffeinated drinks, must be avoided.

When starting diabetes treatment, a healing diet of strict plant-based fresh food (raw food) is required for the first week. Later one-third warm, cooked or baked food can follow, if no further weight reduction is necessary. The recipes marked* should be used only after the diabetic metabolic situation has greatly improved, the body weight has normalised, or type 2 diabetes has been healed. Blood pressure must be down to normal, with no signs of secondary diseases.

Quantity of food

Diet calculations must be based on the severity of the disease.
- rule: small amounts (75 % of diabetics suffer from obesity);
- rule: distribution of harmoniously arranged, small meals throughout the day.

In combination with a new, generally healthy lifestyle with an abundance of pre-midnight sleep, daily hiking and exercise, a good, orderly structure of the day and avoidance of all irritating substances, a wholefood diet rich in fresh foods best meets these two requirements.
With our diet the diabetic will learn relatively easily to avoid excess and poor scheduling of meals, and to find a natural balance. Children, adolescents, and unstable, lean diabetics are a special case. For these, the amount of food must be kept rather high, with careful protection from nervous and climatic stimuli and severe exercise. Their treatment must be continually monitored by a doctor, reviewed and adjusted until the patient gradually reaches a better equilibrium.

Diabetes (i.e. the function of the pancreas) is inseparably connected to the performance of other hormonal glands, particularly the thyroid and the adrenal glands. The diet must take into account all the organs involved. Mental stress or physical trauma or infection may irritate the thyroid or put excessive stress on the adrenal glands, causing diabetes mellitus. Plant-based raw food diet is extremely effective for healing these other hormonal glands too. A high content of secondary plant substances and vitamins – especially vitamins A, B-complex, C, D, E and vitamin B_{12} – must be observed. Chromium and zinc trace elements must be brought into the upper normal range. Often called semi-vitamins, lecithin, inosite and choline, like Omega-3 fatty acids, are important stabilisers of the cell membranes and their "power plants" the mitochondria. They are also of great importance for the proper distribution of lipids in the body and should be abundantly present in food.

The phospholipid lecithin is not only found in yolk, but also in all plants. It is particularly rich in cells of plant seeds and soy beans. Lecithin protects the intestinal wall from bacteria and toxins. It contains poly-unsaturated fatty acids and helps protect cholesterol "packed" in the LDL molecule for transport from its synthesis sites in the liver and intestinal mucosa to the membranes of the cells throughout the body and the myelin of the nerve sheaths of the peripheral and central nervous system. Its polyunsaturated fatty acids are particularly sensitive to oxidative stress, against which the fresh plant-based foods (raw food) is greatly effective.

The adrenal glands weakened by diabetes need an abundance of vitamin C to maintain their function.

Principles of the Bircher-Benner diet and order therapy for diabetics

Total food intake should be reduced to the minimum requirement, but with the highest quality and gentle preparation. Calculated in calories the diet should not exceed 2200 Kcal, but should be low enough to maintain the ideal weight or gradually reduce weight in cases of overweight. Slightly exceeding the calorie intake is not harmful for diabetics, but overfeeding, even to a small extent, is always harmful because caloric overfeeding unnecessarily increases the insulin requirement, even to a small extent, while slight underfeeding of calories lowers it. It must be borne in mind that the calorie calculation is not a qualitative effective food energy, but only a combustion energy. Our diabetes diet is adjusted to the energy potential ordering the biological system in food economy and content so that it contains neither too much nor too little of anything required for the cells and metabolism. As a result, the need for food calculated in calories is considerably lower. See the chapters on food energy and food economics.

Avoid all substances with sugar that passes quickly into the blood: processed sugar, sweet dishes, jam, cakes, candy and honey from bees fed mainly with white sugar (high-quality organic honey may be used sparingly). Also avoid white bread, white pasta, dates and ripe, very sweet fruits. Permitted are wholemeal products, and other fruits and vegetables.

Until diabetes has been cured, the daily amount of food must be distributed in small portions throughout the day. This has the disadvantage that the breaks necessary for healthy peristaltic of the gastrointestinal tract are lost. However, it is necessary in diabetes mellitus, since sudden, high intake of food requires an abundance of insulin, and the liver and muscles must immediately build glycogen from excess sugar to store it. Additionally, excessive carbohydrates must be converted into fat to store it in the fat tissue.

Nutrients should contain 45 % of slowly degradable carbohydrates, 35 % high-quality vegetable fats (lipids with polyunsaturated fatty acids) and 20 % protein. At the beginning, the diet should consist of 100 % plant-based fresh foods (raw food). Later, up to 30 % of cooked whole foods may follow. All irritants should be avoided, as they generate oxidative stress and increase the insulin requirement.

A daily hike of at least one hour is required. If this is not possible due to pain or disabilities, a different type of movement must be found.

Treatment of diabetes mellitus requires an orderly lifestyle, with at least three hours of sleep before midnight. One can easily be active early in the morning. The hormone levels are adjusted to the natural day and the position of the sun. Diabetics often suffer from other hormonal disorders. For example, hypothyroidism occurs in about 15 % of the cases.

Mental health issues have an unfavourable effect on diabetes. Relationship conflicts must be resolved. Fears – captivity in a spider's web of relationship conflicts – hatred and feelings of guilt must be healed. A harmonious lifestyle and a light, cheerful mind are very important for healing.

It is very important that diabetics understand that the diet we teach them is not ours but must become their own. Only then will they succeed in recognising and bearing the necessary responsibility for themselves. We often have an initial tendency to eat beyond what we really need. One must be aware that an excess of food is particularly harmful for diabetics.

Our diet leaves no one hungry. Eating too much is guided by conventional desires. It is important to remember that these desires will soon disappear completely with this diet, and give way to a new, more differentiated sense of taste so that one looks forward to every meal of fresh food. This indicates that a metabolic balance has been achieved. Overweight diabetics experience a slow, steady weight reduction down to the ideal weight. Type 2 diabetics whose insulin levels are still high should remember that weight reduction alone down to ideal weight reduces insulin resistance. Diabetes can heal this way alone, an initial pay-off.

Underweight and juvenile diabetics cannot gain weight with a high-calorie fattening diet. They have usually already tried that. However, weight gain up to one's individual ideal weight is possible with the help of this diet, which is rich in vital substances and is high quality in terms of food economy and energy.

This high-quality composition of the diet is a prerequisite for successful therapy. It is reflected in the blood sugar.

A fasting blood sugar level of 5.6 mmol/l (100 mg%) should be targeted, with no more than 10 mmol/l (180 mg%) one hour after breakfast. Even if these thresholds have not been attained, it is less risky than hypoglycaemia, which is a risk especially for type 1 diabetics or underweight people, or when taking certain antidiabetic drugs. (See the chapter on medical treatment).

Less dangerous hypoglycaemic crises may occur at the beginning of type 2 diabetes, before our diet is started. They happen when patients eat too many easily degradable carbohydrates out of nervousness, fatigue, strong desires or hunger from irritation, causing excessive insulin secretion that temporarily drops the blood sugar level under the standard value until counter-regulation by glucagon begins.

Life order and body training

Patients with diabetes mellitus require a healthy order of life even more than healthy people, in order to create the prerequisite for successful treatment. The sleep and dream phases are biologically specified. Deep, restorative sleep is only possible before midnight. Non-REM (rapid eye movement) sleep phases are unlikely to happen later. There are barely any dreams during these sleep phases. All systems are shut down to rest. After midnight, in the REM phase, dreams have the purpose of healing mental trauma and of giving our consciousness a certain precisely dosed insight into the world of the subconscious. Only the eyes and the diaphragm (to breathe) move during the REM phases. This partial paralysis prevents sleepwalking. Deep restoration of the non-REM phases is extremely important for nocturnal regeneration and healing. Therefore the night's rest should start at 9 p.m. whenever possible. In return, it is possible to get up very early and be active without becoming exhausted.

It is very important to go for a walk of at least half an hour twice a day for physical exercise, and also to go for an evening walk before bed to stimulate the metabolism. It is still generally unknown that scientific studies have shown that steady walking is more effective than strenuous competitive sport in building up one's physical condition. A longer hike should be undertaken regularly at the weekend. It is important to remember that the insulin dose should be reduced before any major exercise (see insulin therapy) or that additional carbohydrate units must be taken. A day hike will save about 20 units of insulin. Medical advice is important for this at first.

Ten minutes of body exercises in the morning and evening with conscious deep breathing are also important.

Swimming or cycling 10 minutes a day should be added in summer, if possible. Diaphragm breathing stimulates the circulation of the upper abdominal organs and therefore the pancreas. One should not spend the entire week sitting down and then go on weekend mountain hikes or strenuous cycling tours, competitions and similar, or force a series of singles tennis or 18-hole golf matches once a week. Daily stamina training 1) exercises the cardiovascular system, muscles, ligaments and tendons; 2) best orders circulation, energy metabolism and the islet cells; and 3) ensures a harmonious use of carbohydrates and order in energy metabolism. This reduces the need for insulin. Sedentary weeks and forced weekend exercise, on the other hand, means lagging and sluggishness alternating with shock-like exhaustion, an increase in blood sugar, followed by a sudden drop. This is stress instead of exercise. Physical training contributes to mental relaxation and well-being.

Hygiene

Hygiene is also part of the diabetic's healthy lifestyle. The skin, as a large protective organ against infection, wounds, hypothermia or overheating, has rich possibilities for adaptation. The capillary system of the skin and its innervation make us aware of dangers from infection and poisoning. Awareness must be practiced specifically with diabetes mellitus. The risk of infections, long-term damage and arteriosclerosis is particularly high. It is very important to wash your hands and feet often, and to care for your nails and teeth carefully. A daily full body shower is important, especially if you have perspired. The roots of the teeth must be carefully examined, and sources of infection removed. Infection foci are dangerous with diabetes. The tonsils must be examined regularly as well. Intestinal rot and constipation must be overcome at all costs, something best achieved by a raw food diet phase of several weeks. The liver and bile ducts require regular examination as well.

Small suppurations must be treated carefully, and cuts must be disinfected and bandaged. Fingernails and toenails must be trimmed very carefully, without injury. Swimming baths are sources of fungal infections for the feet and vagina. Swallowing water while swimming can cause gastrointestinal infections. If you use public baths, treat your feet daily with potassium permanganate or with essential geranium or lavender oil every day. Warm clothing is important in winter to avoid bladder infections. Do not visit people who suffer from catarrh. Frequent chamomile seat baths are necessary for the care of the abdominal organs.

Water applications, stimulation of the circulation, air, light and sun

Daily stimulation of the circulation and the body regulation by a daily alternating shower is very important. Take a very warm, long shower first, until you feel the need to cool off. Then switch the water all the way to cold and rinse your legs, shoulders, face, neck and back and the entire body with cold water. A strong internal warming and blood circulation begins then. It will last for hours.

Many diabetics react particularly well to the Preissnitz body wrap. A sheet is placed in cold water, fully squeezed out and then placed over the entire body in the evening or during the midday rest. It is attached tightly around the body with a flannel tie, so that it soon warms up. The body wrap promotes circulation of the abdominal organs, and consequently the function of the pancreas. It relieves tension, calms the solar plexus and the entire nervous system and is a great help for a restful sleep. Smaller cold-water applications, such as an alternating arm or foot baths, cold thigh gushes, neck gushes, body wraps or partial washes are also helpful to promote body regulation and blood circulation, which is very important in diabetes. One must always make sure to thoroughly warm up before each cold water application (e.g. a hot shower).

Blood circulation can be further stimulated by dry brushing with a soft brush. Walking in the dew and snow is also very effective, though one must be careful to avoid injury.

In the summertime, frequent sunbathing for 20 minutes per body side without sun blocker is important in order not to block out the important UV-B light spectrum. Sunlight causes not only vitamin D_3 synthesis, but has other significant effects so far only partially researched.

Psychological support

Even if the cause of diabetes is mainly physical damage caused in the course of years, decades or even generations, the psyche is still strongly involved in the symptoms.

When type 2 diabetes is recognised early on or during pregnancy, the insulin level is still elevated. This means that the patient is still mainly in the nutrition-based insulin resistance, and the islet cells of the pancreas can still produce additional insulin. At this stage, it is sufficient to carefully explain the nature and causes of diabetes until the patient takes control of his destiny and follows the diet with pleasure and care.

In type 1 diabetes and progressive type 2 diabetes, with the pancreas exhausted, the situation is entirely different. Treatment can still considerably improve the course of the disease, but the disease must be accepted as a personal fate. This is a matter of understanding the danger of secondary diseases and accepting the limitations that prevent them for as long as possible. In doing so, one must learn not to struggle with fate for too long, but to accept it and to look into a positive future in spite of everything. This is done by loving, respecting and honouring one's own life and doing the best one can to stay as healthy as possible. For a diabetic child, the entire family must understand the nature of the disease very well and change their diet to the modern, wholesome, plant-based wholefood diet with a high proportion of raw vegetables that may be new for them. Diabetic camps and schools may help the entire family to understand the nature of the disease, and to learn insulin therapy and calculation of the meals.

Young type 1 diabetics must learn to focus on more important things than gourmandises, fast-food stalls and parties, without becoming resentful.

They need help to realise that, despite their condition, they can become full and valuable members of society. The self-control and maturity acquired by treating their disease may even put them ahead of their peers, and make them role models and helpers to others.

Older diabetics often slip into anxiety and insecurity. They find it difficult to change their habits, which have a certain addictive character, and to discard them in order to bring new, healthy order into their lives, and to take responsibility for themselves and for their family members.

The diagnosis diabetes is always a mental trauma, causing fear of the future, despondency, restlessness and despair. If the nature of the disease and the possibility of taking life into one's own hands is understood, and if the doctor, with all his experience, supports the patient as a friend, the disease can become the starting point for deep reflection on the personal meaning of one's life and relationships. This can lead to an extremely valuable personal maturing progress.

SHORT SUMMARY

Diabetes is a metabolic disorder, a disease of loss. The sugar flows away without fulfilling its function.

Type 1 diabetes: only very partially due to genetic factors
Type 2 diabetes: metabolic diseases caused by incorrect nutrition. At first the insulin level is raised (i.e. insulin resistance), then the insulin-forming cells of the pancreas are exhausted over time.

Diabetics require competent medical treatment. They need knowledge, consistency and insight. Type 2 diabetes can be healed at an early stage, while the insulin level is still elevated. This requires a strict healing diet of 100 % raw food, with a strict order of life, until the insulin resistance is healed and the sugar metabolism has normalised. A seemingly healthy person whose parents suffer from diabetes should have regular check-ups and consider a healthy diet that is predominantly antidiabetic. This book provides an introduction and facilitates the compilation of a diabetes diet for those at risk and those with diabetes.

Eleven basic rules

1. The times of hunger in the two world wars have shown us that the disease diabetes mellitus is significantly reduced by inadequate nutrition. It all but disappeared, in fact. People suffering from hunger do not know diabetes. Diabetes mellitus is a "civilisation disease" of a "wealthy society" that eats too much and the wrong things.

2. It is not only the consumption of sugar that causes diabetes, but overeating in general. Every unnecessarily eaten food is elaborately converted into glucose in the metabolism. This causes an enormous strain on the metabolism by depositing degenerative metabolic slags in the intercellular substance of the entire body, along with oxidative stress. All of this produces the entire range of continually growing degenerative "civilisation diseases". Diabetics need to eat small quantities of whole foods of energetic high quality. These are provided by plant-based whole foods with a high share of living plant foods (raw food) containing high energy potential and food economy, as well as high content of vital substances and secondary plant substances (phytochemicals).

3. In the early stages diabetics tend to be overweight from overeating and lack of exercise. This overloads not only the pancreas but the entire organism: heart, blood vessels, kidneys, liver and nervous system. The diet described in this book can relieve the metabolism and heal the patient. This way type 2 diabetes in the hyperinsulinism stage due to insulin resistance is able to heal. Later, or with type 1 diabetes, the course can be influenced very positively, and most secondary diseases can be avoided.

4. Fresh plant-based food, including acidic fruit, cause a base excess in the metabolism.

5. The diabetic organism is prone to hyperacidity. More than any other sick person, the diabetic needs a diet rich in bases, with plenty of fruit and vegetables, and a high proportion of raw vegetables.

6. Denaturated carbohydrates (e.g. white sugar or white-flour products) are resorbed very quickly, and demand rapid and very high insulin excretion by the pancreas. The diabetic organism will be unable to master this "stress situation", leaving the sugars in the blood and letting them flow into the urine instead of providing them to the cells. Whole (i.e. non-denaturated or peeled) carbohydrates, as they are contained in vegetables, fruit and wholemeal cereals, are broken down much more slowly. The blood sugar level rises much more slowly, and the peak is flatter. They contain mostly sugar types that do not require insulin to be used. This protects the islet cells in the pancreas. The diabetic needs carbohydrates but must limit himself to whole, non-denaturated ones. Denatured, sugar and white-flour products must be avoided entirely.

7. Fats and proteins must always have the right proportion to each other in the diet. Otherwise they cannot be utilised and will cause massive over-acidification from metabolic slags, which cause massive damage to all organs. This puts the diabetic at risk for long-term damage and premature aging.

8. Diabetics must take special care to consume food rich in enzymes and vital substances. A diet of fresh vegetable foods fulfils these conditions best and corresponds most closely to the requirements of food economy. The patient will not eat too little or too much of anything.

9. Shock, excessive strain, stress, acute diseases, accidents, fears, sorrow, anxiety and insecurity, humiliation, anger, fury and hate may cause the metabolism to become unbalanced in diabetes mellitus. The diabetic must learn to recognise the danger of such situations and to actively confront them before they become dangerous for their health. In such stressful situations, he must adhere to our diet and the new, healthy order of life particularly strictly. Febrile diseases require bed rest and medical care. Diabetics need a life that is as regular as possible. They must mature under their illness.

10. Suppurations, intestinal rot and focal infections (tonsils, teeth, gall bladder) can worsen diabetes as additional strains. Focal infections must be healed, and chronic constipation must be overcome by a healing diet rich in raw-food. The teeth must be carefully cleaned after every meal, the gums massaged, the skin protected from infections with careful care, in addition to dry brushing, alternating washes, strict cleanliness and careful foot care. Injuries must always be carefully disinfected and bandaged immediately. An annual medical and dental check-up is absolutely necessary.

11. Physical exercise and breathing increase the activity of the metabolism. This lowers the blood sugar level and allows better utilisation of sugar. Physical training increases the ability to produce insulin, as the circulation in the abdominal organs is activated as well. The diabetic must perform daily gymnastics, hikes and deep breathing in fresh air; he should go to bed early and get up early, and avoid lack of sleep and exhaustion.

THE BIRCHER-BENNER DIABETES DIET

General information

As already described in detail, type 2 diabetes is caused by insulin resistance for an extended period. The islet cells of the pancreas produce excessive insulin levels until they are exhausted. At this early stage, the disease is curable by strict diet of pure plant-based raw foods over several weeks. When the glucose stress test, insulin level and body weight have normalised, healing can be confirmed. To prevent a relapse the raw vegetable portion of the diet should remain at two-thirds after this. Foods with a deep glycaemic index and a low glycaemic charge should still be preferred after healing. Even then, it is worth returning every now and then to phases of a strict raw food diet for one or more weeks.

Unfortunately neither type 2 diabetes, in which the insulin level has already dropped, nor type 1 diabetes can be healed. However, phases of a strict raw food diet are a great help, as they are intended to prevent secondary diseases. Cooked food should have the lowest possible glycaemic index and a low glycaemic charge. It should not exceed one-third of the total food quantity.

The Bircher-Benner Manual No. 4 on fresh juices, raw vegetable and fruit dishes provides very important information on the effects of the raw food diet on diabetics and on the prevention of secondary diseases.

The levels of vitamins B_{12} and D_3 should be checked every six months. They must be kept in the upper normal range.

DIET RECIPES FOR DIABETICS

General information

Legend
Gram = g
Calories = K (caloric value)
Protein = E*
Fat = F*
Carbohydrates = CH*
Bread units = BU (12 g CH = 1 BU)

(* in grams)

Bread units and their calculation

The calculation in bread units has proven its worth for everyday use.
Remember: 12 g CH (carbohydrates) = 1 BU (bread unit)
Bread units are used in diabetes that must BU treated with insulin to estimate the necessary insulin dose before the meal. To calculate precisely, one can use "gram carbohydrates". For those used to **"bread units"**, their calculations are always given in brackets. However, these are approximate and have been slightly rounded up or down to keep them within a practicable framework, e.g.
one bread unit corresponds to 12 g carbohydrates.

The following rough calculations can be made:
3 to 9 g CH = ½ BU
From 9 to 15 g CH = 1 BU
From 15 to 21 g CH = 1½ BU
From 21 to 27 g CH = 2 BU etc.

The carbohydrate unit

Carbohydrate units are sometimes used instead of bread units.
1 carbohydrate unit corresponds to 10 g carbohydrates.

Sugar in the diet

Diabetics should avoid sugar, especially processed sugar, which enters the blood far too quickly and therefore increases the blood sugar level. To sweeten dishes we recommend fructose or sorbitol, the sugar obtained from rowan berries. These two types of sugar produce a very small increase in blood sugar. They must be used sparingly, however. Diabetics who are mildly affected may use high-quality honey or fruit concentrate in small quantities from time to time.

The recipe section contains a great many tasty recipes, so there is no lack of enjoyment from food. However, depending on the stage of the disease and any secondary diseases that have already occurred, the prescriptions must be selected. It is worthwhile for every diabetic to read the Bircher-Benner Manual No. 19 for patients with hypertension, cardiovascular disease and arteriosclerosis in order to learn more about the prevention of the secondary diseases of diabetes.

Recipe section

Recipes marked * must only be prepared for the preventive diet due to genetic predisposition, or after type 2 diabetes has healed. They are only allowed after normalisation of body weight and in the absence of any signs of secondary disease.

Recipes for fresh plant-based foods (raw food)

The Bircher müesli

The Bircher müesli, as first introduced by Dr. Bircher, has remained the most tried-and-tested and best food diet based on our many years of experience. In principle, sour, white-fleshed, juicy apples are the best (e.g. Kläräpfel, Gravensteiner, Sauergrauch, Menznauer-Jäger, Jonathan, Ontario, Wellington, Glockenäpfel, Champagner-Reinetten, Topaz, possibly Bonäpfel and Granny Smith apple).

If apples that are dry or have little taste must be used in the late season, their aroma can be enriched by adding oranges cut into small pieces. Add 1 teaspoon of cold-pressed linseed oil, if available.

1. Bircher müesli with almond puree
8 g fine oat flakes or millet flakes, fresh ground (opt.)
50 g cold water
8 g lemon juice
10 g almond puree
12 g fruit concentrate, fructose or sorbitol (if almond puree is too mushy and apples slightly dry, add 20–25 g water)
200 g apples
8 g rice germ or wheat germ, or germinated wheat grains

Soak the flakes for 12 hours if possible. Mix everything well with a whisk. Wash, dry with a clean cloth, remove stalks and flowers. Grate the apples directly into the sauce with the Bircher grater. Stir frequently so that they do not turn brown. Instead of grating, the apples can also be cut into small pieces and worked in with a hand blender. Grate shortly before serving.
K = 239 E = 4.5 g F = 6 g CH = 40 g (= 3 BU)

2. Bircher müesli with yoghurt
8 g oat flakes
50 g water
10 g yoghurt
8 g lemon juice
12 g fruit concentrate or honey
200 g apples
6 g hazelnuts or almonds, ground

Soak for 12 hours.
Mix to form a smooth sauce.
Prepare like recipe no. 1.
Sprinkle the prepared dish with ground almonds.
K = 194 E = 3 g F = 4 g CH = 35 g (= 3 BU)

3. Bircher müesli with cream*
8 g oat flakes
30 g water
30 g fresh, non-UHT-processed cream
8 g lemon juice
12 g fruit concentrate or honey
200 g apples
6 g hazelnuts or almonds, ground

Soak for 12 hours.

Beat slightly and mix with the lemon juice and fruit concentrate.
Prepare like recipe no. 1.
Sprinkle over the prepared dish.
K = 260 E = 4 g F = 11 g CH = 36 g (= 3 BU)

4. Müesli with berries or stone fruit
Particularly high vitamin C content
Prepare the sauce as in recipe no. 1
150–200 g strawberries,
washed and selected
or
raspberries, rinsed
blueberries
currants
blackberries
peaches
apricots
oranges

Crush with a wooden pestle or fork. Run through a chrome-plated chopper or food mil, or cut finely with a knife. These fruits have approximately the same values as apples.

5. Bircher müesli with various fruits
Prepare the sauce as in recipe no. 1.
strawberries and raspberries
strawberries, raspberries and currants
strawberries and apples
blackberries and apples
apples with finely cut orange and tangerine pieces
peaches or apricots, etc.
Thoroughly mix the fruits into the sauce.

Raw vegetables and salads

The following four basic rules should be observed when preparing raw vegetables:

1. Fresh and good quality
Organic vegetables are best, if possible from one's own garden.
Raw vegetables should be prepared as close to consumption as possible, so that no withering and leaking of the juice is possible, and so the crushed food is only briefly exposed to oxygen (air). It is important to mix the vegetables quickly with the dressing.

2. Thorough cleaning
The following rules on the cleaning of vegetables must be observed in order to prevent worming and infection by coli bacteria. Biologically grown vegetables without manure fertilisation contain no worm eggs.

2a. Cleaning leafy vegetables
Head lettuce, endive/chicory, lettuce, white cabbage, cabbage, red cabbage etc.: Separate the leaves, remove brown and damaged areas, and leave in salt water for 15 min (1 handful salt to 5 l water) if germ infestation is suspected, especially in tropical and subtropical countries.

Rinse repeatedly. Preferably rinse each leaf individually under a water shower or jet. Dry in a wire basket, salad swing or clean cloth. Field and cut lettuces, spinach, dandelion, cress, Brussels sprouts and similar small-leaved lettuces require special care in cleaning and washing. Rinse small portions repeatedly, and remove roots and tough stems.
Cut white or red chicory in half, remove outermost leaves and rinse well.

2b. Cleaning root vegetables
Clean celery (celeriac), carrots, black salsify, beetroot (red beet), radish, kohlrabi and radishes with a brush under running water; peel and immediately place in cold water with salt and lemon juice (½ lemon or pressed lemon peel in 5 l water) so that the vegetables do not lose their fresh colour.

2c. Cleaning vegetable fruits
Tomatoes, cucumbers, courgettes, peppers. Wash the fruits first, then peel or chop them as necessary. Peel cucumbers from the middle outwards, cutting off the bitter

ends. Tender cucumbers can also be used unpeeled.
Only use young, tender courgettes for salads. Do not peel them. Cut the peppers in half and remove the seeds, cut them into thick pieces and, if necessary, soak them in water if they are too spicy.
Cauliflower, celery, leek, fennel:
Cauliflower: cut into larger pieces, cut away damaged parts, peel the stalk slightly and soak in salted water.
Stalk celery: wash, peel, cut away hard parts.
Leek: halve, clean and rinse under the tap set to shower.
Fennel: halve and wash.

2d. Special cleaning methods
If there is any doubt that vegetables and fruits are germ-free and clean (especially in southern and tropical countries and when using manure fertilisation), observe the following cleaning methods:
1. To remove worm eggs and vermin, place the vegetables in diluted saline solution (1 handful salt for 5 l water). The saline solution will dislodge worm eggs attached by a protein layer, so that the vegetables are free of them when thoroughly rinsed again.
2. Bacteria (e.g. coli bacteria and fungi) can be removed with citric acid or vinegar. Prepare a solution of 60 g citric acid (available in drugstores) in 1 l of water and leave the vegetables, particularly leafy ones, in this solution for 15 min. Then rinse thoroughly under running water. Filter and store the citric acid solution. It can be used three or four times.
3. Bulbs and fruit vegetables can be filtered after cleaning and washing, and submersed in boiling water for 10 seconds. The outer layer becomes germ-free while the vegetables remain raw inside.
4. Even without these preparations, vegetable and fruit juices become almost sterile by adding squeezed lemon juice (i.e. one-fifth of the juice) to them.
5. To protect from amoeba in the tropics, submerse the pre-cleaned vegetables in a chlorinated lime solution (5 g chlorinated lime for 1 l water). Then wash with boiled water, which removes the chlorinated lime entirely.

3. Harmonious composition
Every raw vegetable dish should contain all three types of vegetables – root, fruit and leaf – if at all possible, so that the contents complement each other in each meal. The green leaf should not be missing, especially in food for people who are sick. Variety can be added with dressings. The triad of colours enhances the beauty of the platter and contributes to the pleasure of eating.
Small garnishes of herbs, radishes, young carrots etc. can make the raw vegetable platter more colourful and festive for special occasions. However, the triad of raw vegetables per meal should not be exceeded on a regular basis. Variety over the course of the day is to be preferred. Excessive variety is not good for digestion.

4. Chopping the various vegetable types
Head lettuce, lettuce, lamb's lettuce, dandelion, cress
lettuce, endive, chicory
spinach, leek, celery stalks
white cabbage, red cabbage
carrot, celery (celeriac), beetroot, radish, black salsify, kohlrabi
cucumbers, courgettes, radishes, cauliflower
– leave whole or halve the larger leaves.
– cut into strips ½ cm wide.
– cut into very fine strips.
– grate finely.
– grate with a Bircher grater or a coarser grater.
– grate into fine slices.
– grate finely the cauliflower blossom and tender stalk parts.

Dressings for raw vegetables and salads

6. Oil dressing
Only cold-pressed vegetable oils of biological quality should be used. Olive oil and sunflower oil should be supplemented with ⅓ linseed oil, as their content in omega-3 fatty acids is too low.

For 1 portion:
8 g oil
2 g lemon juice
onion, garlic (opt.)
2 g fresh or 1 knife tip
of dried herbs
Mix well.
K = 74 E = – F = 8 g CH = – 0 g (= 0 BU)

7. Mayonnaise dressing, for 4 portions*
15 g yolk, whisked
150 g oil
a few drops of lemon juice
(1 yolk is enough for 6–8 portions)
Add oil to the yolk drop by drop while stirring evenly with a whisk.
K = 1440 E = 2 g F = 154 g CH = – 0 g
(= 0 BU)
For 1 portion:
10 g mayonnaise
2 g lemon juice
onion, garlic (opt.)
2 g fresh or
1 knife tip of dried herbs
= 14 g mayonnaise:
K = 90 E = 0,1 g F = 10 g CH = – 0 g (= 0 BU)

8. Mayonnaise dressing with soy flour instead of egg, for 4 portions
15 soy flour
100 g water
200 g oil
10 g lemon juice
Mix to a smooth batter.
Add alternatingly while stirring slowly and constantly with a whisk.

For 1 portion:
10 g mayonnaise
2 g lemon juice
onion, garlic (opt.)
2 g fresh or 1 knife tip of dried herbs
= 14 g mayonnaise
Mix all ingredients well.
K = 90 E = 0,1 g F = 10 g CH = – 0 g
(= 0 BU)

9. Cream dressing, for 1 portion*
20 g cream
5 g quark
2 g lemon juice
onion, garlic (opt.)
1 g fresh or 1 knife tip of dried herbs
Mix well with a whisk.
K = 54 E = 2 g F = 5 g CH = 1 g (= 0 BU)

10. Yoghurt dressing, for 1 portion
30 g yoghurt
a few drops of lemon juice
onion, garlic (opt.)
1 g fresh or 1 knife tip of dried herbs
K = 20 E = 1 g F = 1 g CH = 2 g (= 0 BU)

Not every dressing is suitable for every raw vegetable. The following has proved a good approach:

The following salads and raw vegetables		are prepared with:
11. Head lettuce	do not chop (whole leaves)	Oil dressing, chives, onions
12. Cut lettuce	uncut	Oil dressing, chives, onions
13. Endives	cut in strips of 1 cm	Oil dressing or mayonnaise, chives, onions, parsley
14. Lettuce	cut in strips of 1 cm	Oil dressing or mayonnaise, basil, marjoram
15. Lamb's lettuce	uncut	Oil dressing or mayonnaise, onions

The following salads and raw vegetables		are prepared with:
16. Cress	uncut	Oil dressing or mayonnaise, onions
17. Spinach	cut strips ½ cm wide	Oil dressing or mayonnaise, peppermint
18. Cabbage salads: White cabbage Sauerkraut Brussels sprouts Savoy cabbage Chinese cabbage	slice, cut into thin pieces	Oil dressing or mayonnaise, lovage, savory, thyme, cumin
19. Tomatoes	slice or dice	Oil dressing or mayonnaise, basil, thyme, dill
20. Cucumbers	slice	Oil dressing or mayonnaise, dill
21. Fennel	finely cut with knife and cut with chopping knife	Oil dressing or mayonnaise, onions, chives
22. Bell pepper	cut fine strips	Oil dressing or mayonnaise, chives
23. Radish	slice or grate	Oil dressing or cream dressing, chives
24. Radishes	slice	Oil dressing or cream dressing, chives
25. Stalk celery	cut finely	Oil dressing or cream dressing, onions, chives
26. Courgettes	slice or grate coarsely	Oil dressing or mayonnaise, dill, basil
27. Carrots	grate finely	Cream dressing or oil dressing, marjoram, lovage
28. Celery	grate finely	Cream dressing or mayonnaise, basil, thyme
29. Beetroot	grate finely or coarsely	Cream dressing or mayonnaise, lovage, thyme, cumin
30. Cauliflower	cut off florets closely, finely grate stems	Cream dressing or mayonnaise, basil, marjoram, walnuts
31. Chicory	cut in strips of 1 cm	Cream dressing or oil dressing, tarragon, marjoram
32. Jerusalem artichoke	grate	Cream dressing, thyme, balm
33. Kohlrabi	slice and chop with chopping knife or grate	Cream dressing or oil dressing, thyme, lovage
34. Red cabbage	slice or cut finely	Cream dressing or oil dressing, a small number of grated apples, caraway, lovage

Chives, parsley and onions can be added (moderately) to any raw vegetables.

Sauerkraut

Sauerkraut is a particularly valuable raw vegetable, especially in winter. It is more easily digestible raw than cooked. In the preparation of steamed sauerkraut, taste and digestibility can be improved by adding finely chopped fresh food sauerkraut.

35. Sauerkraut salad

Sauerkraut is separated and chopped, and mixed with a few caraway seeds (or ground caraway), 3 to 4 cut juniper berries, finely chopped onion and an apple cut into small strips. Drizzle everything with the juice of a lemon and two tablespoons of olive oil. Field salad and any raw vegetables from root vegetables are recommended as a supplement.

Fresh cereals

36. Sprouted cereal grains
Particularly high content of vitamin E and B groups. General strengthening. Wheat, rye, oats, barley (wholemeal types). Buy grains that germinate easily. No pickled seeds!

1st day	evening:	wash the grains on a screen under running water, put them into a bowl. Cover with water, keep at room temperature, close to the oven.
2nd day	morning:	rinse the grains and spread dry on a flat plate at room temperature, close to the oven
	evening:	put into bowl and cover with water. Keep at room temperature, close to the oven
3rd day	morning:	rinse the grains and spread dry on the plate.
	evening:	put into bowl and cover with a damp cloth, keep at room temperature, close to the oven, until the grains have developed 1 to 2 cm long sprouts.

1 tablespoon of germinated grain is used per meal, up to maximum 2 tablespoons per day.

Table II: Nutritional composition of some fresh juices

	100 g of juice contain:				
	K	E g	F g	CH g	BU
1. Fruit juices					
Apple juice	47	0.1	–	11	1
Elderberry juice	38	2	–	8	½
Grape juice	74	0.3	–	18	1½
Sea buckthorn berry juice	26	0.9	2.3	–	–
Orange juice	47	0.8	0.3	10	1
Grapefruit juice	28	0.6	0.1	9	1
Tangerine juice	43	0.9	0.3	9	1
Lemon juice	24	0.3	0.1	8	½
Coconut milk	22	0.3	0.4	4	½
Acerola concentrate (powdered)	263	5.6	1.2	58	5
2. Vegetable juices					
Carrot juice	27	0.6	–	6	½
Tomato juice	22	1.0	0.2	4	½
Beetroot juice	42	1/1	–	10	1
Spinach juice	13	1.4	–	2	–

(Beetroot = red beet)

Fresh juices

37. Fruit juices
Serve immediately after pressing. Waiting reduces value.
Additions as desired or required: lemon juice, fruit concentrate, sea buckthorn, cream, yoghurt, almond milk, linseed, $1/3$ rice or barley gruel (for sensitive stomach or gastrointestinal disease).

a) *Unmixed fruit juices*
(without any addition)
oranges, tangerines, grapefruits, apples, pears, strawberries, blueberries, currants, raspberries, peaches, apricots, plums

b) *Mixed fruit juices*
e.g. orange juice, tangerine juice, grapefruit juice, persimmon juice or berry juice with apple juice (opt.), or
berry juice with peach, apricot or plum juice (opt.).

38. Vegetable juices
Drink fresh: high content of minerals, vitamins and secondary plant substances. Each juice has its own special value (see chapter on minerals and vitamins and on the secondary plant substances that are particularly effective against diabetes).

a) *Unmixed vegetable juices*
Tomatoes, carrots, red beets, radish, cabbage, celery, potatoes, all leaf, tuber and root vegetables.

b) *Mixed vegetable juices*
According to our experience, mixtures that have proven themselves are particularly successful are:
Carrots, tomatoes, spinach (equal parts)
Tomatoes and carrots
Tomatoes and spinach
Other mixes (and cocktails) can be combined as desired. The earthy taste of root vegetables can be pleasantly brightened by adding sun-ripened fruit.

For diversity, add sorrel, stinging nettle, chives, parsley, onions, tender celery leaves or bulbs and other herbs before pressing.
Additions per glass (1½ to 2 dl): 10 g cream, a little lemon juice, fruit concentrate (opt.), linseed (opt.), rice or barley gruel for patients with gastrointestinal issues.
Other leafy vegetables or salads can also be used (e.g. dandelion, white cabbage, cabbage, head lettuce, endive, lamb's lettuce, lettuce). In spring for blood cleansing treatment with stinging nettle, sorrel and dandelion juice.

Plant milk types

39. Almond milk
10 g almond puree
4 g fruit concentrate
1½ dl water
(1½ dl water and ½ dl fruit juice cause slight thickening)
Mix almond puree and fruit concentrate with the whisk and add the water drop by drop. (Hint: add the water immediately and stir with a blender, which makes the milk pleasantly frothy.)
K = 76 E = 2 g F = 5 g CH = 6 g (= ½ BU)

40. Almond milk of fresh almonds
(very easy to digest)
15 g almonds, peeled
(no bitter almonds!)
4 g fructose powder
1½ dl water
Mix in blender, strain if necessary.
K = 76 E = 2 g F = 5 g CH = 6 g (= ½ BU)

41. Pine nut milk
15 g pine seeds, washed
4 g fruit concentrate
1½ dl water
Prepare like almond milk.
K = 76 E = 2 g F = 5 g CH = 6 g (= ½ BU)

42. Sesame milk
(rich in biologically high-quality fatty acids)
2 dl water (cold or warm, depending on taste)
15 g Helva purée
2 g lemon juice
4 g fruit concentrate
Mix Helva purée and fruit concentrate with the whisk and add water drop by drop.
Particularly tasty with fresh banana and stirred with a blender.
$K = 76$ $E = 2$ g $F = 5$ g $CH = 6$ g $(= ½ BU)$

43. Sesame cream
Like sesame milk, but with less water added
For cold dishes, and as a substitute for cream.
$K = 76$ $E = 2$ g $F = 5$ g $CH = 6$ g $(= ½ BU)$

44. Sesame frappé
Like sesame milk or sesame cream with added fruit juice, grape juice etc.
$K = 76$ $E = 2$ g $F = 5$ g $CH = 6$ g $(= ½ BU)$

45. Soy milk (Molat)
10 g Molat (3 level teaspoons)
1 dl water
3 tablespoons orange juice
Whisk.
$K = 70$ $E = 2$ g $F = 2$ g $CH = 10$ g $(= 1 BU)$

Hot food

The information on cooking times in the recipes is for conventional cooking. A pressure cooker or a steamer would be preferable, because preparation with them is much gentler and the nutritional values are better preserved. The preparation times are then reduced to about one-fifth of the conventional cooking time. Onions can be pre-sautéed separately and added before cooking.

Butter, health-food store vegetable fats and oils

46. We recommend:
Fresh butter
to refine the dishes and in most recipes of the diet forms. A little is added when preparing the dish on the plate.

Health-food-store vegetable fat
vegetable fat emulsions from naturally solid fats such as coconut oil or palm kernel oil in combination with the highest possible proportion of liquid oils and germ oils. Under no circumstances may they contain hydrogenated vegetable oils.

Nut and almond paste
very fine, nutty taste, versatile use in kitchen and at the table, can be used as bland diet, also in place of fresh butter with vegetables, potatoes, rice.

Sunflower oil
Corn oil
Linseed oil
Olive oil
cold pressed and biologically gently treated, very valuable for its purity as a fat and healthier for most people, as well as easily digestible. Linseed oil, safflower oil, rapeseed oil and other oils with a higher content of polyunsaturated fatty acids (omega-3 and omega-6) are not suitable for heating above body temperature. Olive oil contains almost only monounsaturated fatty acids and is therefore suitable for heating up to 170 °C. It is easier to digest than heated butter.

NB: For health food cuisine, other organic, gently processed vegetable fats and oils from the health-food store are also recommended.
Vegetable oils with polyunsaturated fatty acids must be stored in a cool, dark place. The proportion of oil containing omega-3 must be at least one-fifth in relation to omega-6; a higher ratio is preferred. Lin-

seed oil contains approx. 60 % omega-3 fatty acids. It can be added to Bircher müesli and salad dressings (approx. ⅓), or 1 to 2 tablespoons can be taken 3 times per day with each meal.
Linseed oil is very easily digestible and does not cause weight gain. Our manuals no. 19 and no. 4 will tell you more about the great importance of oils and fatty acids.

Soups

For recipes of over 250 calories, halve the amounts.
Except for the vegetable broth, which is calculated for two to three days, the soups are calculated for one portion. In a small household, where fresh vegetable broth cannot be prepared daily, ordinary water can be used, with a biological health-food store yeast extract liquid or paste or vegetarian bouillon cubes used as a taste additive. Make sure that no flavour enhancers (e.g. glutamate) are contained.
Cream improves every soup and every vegetable, but milk can usually be used instead of cream. Rice milk, which is available in organic quality in many places today, is also very suitable for refinement.
Health-food store yeast extract is a very rich vitamin-B yeast product (rich in glutathione and lecithin). Salt-free yeast extract, which is very important for high blood pressure, is also available in health-food stores.

47. Vegetable broth (for 4 portions)
Choose the vegetables according to the season (e.g. celery, beets, certain cabbage or kohlrabi, leeks, tomatoes and onions). Hard but healthy vegetable parts can be used as well as potato peels etc.
10 g olive oil or health-food store vegetable fat
1 onion
2 carrots

1 small celery (celeriac)
cabbage, chard leaves
1 leek stem
1–1½ l water, cold, with lovage, basil or other fresh or dried herbs
½ laurel leaf

Halve the onion with the brown peel and roast the cut area until brown.
Cut the vegetables into small pieces, add and cook for at least 30 min, covered and at low heat.
Add water and cook for 2 hours at low heat. Season to taste.
K = 77 E = – F = 8 g CH = 0 g
(0 BU)

48. Vegetable bouillon (for 1 portion)
2½ dl (approximately) vegetable broth
poss. health-food store yeast extract (opt.)
5 g butter, fresh

Serve the hot vegetable broth on butter and herbs.
Season with: Parsley, chives, freshly chopped herbs
K = 56 E = – F = 6 g CH = 0 g
(0 BU)

Soup add-ins

49. Egg custard*
1 small egg
very little salt
75 g milk (1½ dl)
nutmeg, ground

Beat the egg with a pinch of salt, add the warm milk and continue beating. Place in a buttered casserole dish or in cups and simmer in a covered water bath for 25–30 min until the mixture is firm. Turn over the cooled egg mixture and cut into small cubes.
K = 121 E = 8 g F = 8 g CH = 4 g
(0 BU)

50. Semolina dumplings*
10 g butter
10 g fine semolina
½–1 egg
200 g vegetable broth (= 2 dl)

Stir until fluffy.
Mix well with the butter and let rest for ½ hour. Use a teaspoon to shape dumplings; place them in the boiling vegetable broth and let steep slightly for 15–20 min.
Season with: marjoram, nutmeg
K = 200 E = 7 g F = 15 g CH = 8 g (= ½ BU)

51. Gold cubes*
25 g wholemeal bread
½–1 egg, whisked
10–20 g milk
5 g olive oil or health-food store vegetable fat

Cut into even cubes.
Mix, pour on and wait until it is absorbed.
Bake the cubes in it until golden yellow.
K = 173 E = 8 g F = 9 g CH = 12 g (= 1 BU)

52. Sago soup with vegetable add-ins
(Sago starch is a taste-neutral thickening agent made from granulated starch produced from the marrow of the trunk of the true sago palm)
10 g sago
500 g vegetable broth
5 g olive oil or health-food store vegetable fat
30 g carrots, cut into small cubes
30 g celery (celeriac), finely diced
30 g leek, fine stripes

Stir into the boiling vegetable broth.
Sauté thoroughly, add to vegetable broth and cook for ½ hour, then place in soup bowl.
Season with: Phag, health-food store yeast extract, parsley, soup green, chives (add to soup bowl).
K = 123 E = 1 g F = 8 g CH = 11 g (= 1 BU)

NB: The vegetables can also all be cut into fine strips, as for Julienne soup.

53. Rice soup, clear
5 g olive oil or health-food store vegetable fat
¼ onion, chopped
20 g carrots
20 g celery (celeriac)
25 g leek
10 g rice
500 g vegetable broth, hot, chives

Sauté ingredients.
Add vegetable broth and cook for 15–20 min.
Pour into the soup bowl.
K = 145 E = 2 g F = 9 g CH = 14 g (= 1 BU)

54. Rice soup, italian style
5 g olive oil or health-food store vegetable fat
60 g vegetables, finely diced (carrots, onions, celery stalks)
100 g spinach, finely chopped
15 g rice
500 g water
5 g butter
10 g cheese, finely grated

Sauté ingredients until the vegetables have taken on colour and the juice is reduced.
Add water and butter and cook for 20 min.
Pour into soup bowl.
Sprinkle the cheese.
K = 214 E = 7 g F = 8 g CH = 18 g (= 1½ BU)

55. Soy soup
5 g olive oil or health-food store vegetable fat
20 g onion, chopped
10 g soy flour
50 g tomatoes, peeled and diced
500 g vegetable broth
pinch of salt

Sauté ingredients.
Add vegetable broth slowly.

Cook for ¼ hour.
K=138 E=4 g F=10 g CH=6 g (=½ BU)

56. Gruel soup
20 g oat flakes
500 g water, salt (opt.)
10 g cream

Boil, cook for 30–40 min, then strain.
Add cream for flavour.
K=81 E=2 g F=3 g CH=11 g (=1 BU)

57. Tomato soup, 1st option
10 g olive oil or health-food store vegetable fat
onion
20 g carrots
40 g celery (celeriac)
25 g leek
garlic clove
rosemary
100 g tomatoes
500 g vegetable broth
tomato puree if desired
5 g butter or
10 g cream
chives

Heat oil or vegetable fat, then cut everything into small pieces and sauté in the health-food store vegetable fat.
Add butter or cream and chives, cook for ½ hour and then strain.
Pour into the soup bowl.
Finely chop and add chives.
K=197 E=2 g F=15 g CH=11 g (=1 BU)

58. Tomato soup, 2nd option*
200 g summer tomatoes, ripe
2 g lemon juice or
20 g cream

Cut into pieces, boil briefly, strain, and serve the soup lukewarm or cold.
K=88 E=3 g F=5 g CH=7 g (= ½ BU)

59. Carrot soup
5 g olive oil or health-store vegetable fat
onion

40 g carrot, sliced
500 g vegetable broth
100 g milk
5 g caraway
10 g cream

Sauté.
Add, cook for ½ hour, strain.
Combine.
Pour into soup bowl.
Season with: Celery herb or lovage – or marjoram.
K=182 E=3 g F=14 g CH=9 g (=1 BU)

60. Spinach or chard soup
5 g olive oil or health-food store vegetable fat
onion
½ garlic clove
10 g soy flour
500 g vegetable broth
5 g milk
50 g spinach
10 g cream

Sauté.
Add and cook for 20 min.
Mix finely chopped spinach and add to the soup. Let the mixture simmer.
Pour into soup bowl.
Season with: nutmeg, parsley, chives, health-food store yeast extract, sage leaves (opt.).
K=182 E=3 g F=14 g CH=9 g (=1 BU)

61. Cauliflower soup
5 g olive oil or health-food store vegetable fat
10 g soy flour
100 g cauliflower
500 g vegetable broth
tip of laurel leaf
a little basil
cauliflower florets
10 g cream

Sauté.
Cook florets separately.

Cut the stalk into small pieces and sauté briefly.
Add, cook for ¾ hours and strain.
Pour into soup bowl.
Add for refinement.
K = 182 E = 3 g F = 14 g CH = 9 g (= 1 BU)

62. Celery soup
5 g olive oil or health-food store vegetable fat
with ½ onion, chopped
60 g celery (celeriac), cut into small pieces
12 g soy flour
500 g vegetable broth
¼ laurel leaf
lovage
10 g cream

Sauté.
Sprinkle over, sauté.
Add, cook for ¾ hours.
Pour into soup bowl.
K = 182 E = 3 g F = 14 g CH = 9 g (= 1 BU)

63. Chervil soup
5 g olive oil or health-store vegetable fat
onion
60 g potatoes, diced
5 g soy flour
500 g vegetable broth
5 g chervil, chopped
5 g cream

Sauté.
Add, cook for ½ hours and strain.
Pour into soup bowl.
K = 182 E = 3 g F = 14 g CH = 9 g (= 1 BU)

64. Spring soup
5 g olive oil or health-food store vegetable fat
10 g soy flour
500 g water or vegetable broth
onion
10 g spinach leaves
tender carrots
50 g milk
10 g cream

Sauté briefly.
Add, cook for ½ hour.
Finely chop the spinach leaves and add to the soup.
Pour into soup bowl.
Season with: lovage, sorrel, nettle or dandelion leaves.
K = 182 E = 3 g F = 14 g CH = 9 g (= 1 BU)

65. Potato soup
5 g olive oil or health-food store vegetable fat
20 g leek
30 g celery
30 g carrots
100 g potatoes, chopped
5 g soy flour
500 g vegetable broth
marjoram
10 g cream
chives

Sauté thoroughly.
Sprinkle over.
Add, cook for ½ hour and strain.
Pour into soup bowl.
Sprinkle over.
K = 234 E = 5 g F = 12 g CH = 25 g (= 2 BU)

66. Potato soup with leeks
5 g olive oil or health-food store vegetable fat
50 g leeks, cut into fine strips
8 g soy flour
500 g vegetable broth
60 g potatoes, chopped
5–10 g cream

Sauté thoroughly.
Sprinkle over.
Add.
Add and cook until soft.
Pour into soup bowl.
Season with: health-store yeast extract, basil, marjoram, dried porcini mushrooms.
K = 207 E = 5 g F = 13 g CH = 17 g (1½ BU)

67. Potato soup with soy flour
12 g soy flour
500 g vegetable broth
60 g potatoes, chopped
pinch of salt
caraway, marjoram (opt.)
10 g cheese, grated
10 g cream

Roast and pour on.
Add and cook until soft.
Pour into soup bowl.
K = 207 E = 8 g F = 12 g CH = 15 g
(= 1½ BU)

68. Cabbage soup with potatoes
5 g olive oil or health-food store
vegetable fat
onion
80 g cabbage, finely chopped
5 g soy flour
50 g potatoes, sliced
500 g water
pinch of salt
10 g cream

Cook until cabbage softens.
Sprinkle and sauté briefly.
Add and cook for ½ hour.
Pour into soup bowl.
Season with: dill or caraway.
K = 149 E = 4 g F = 8 g CH = 15 g (= 1½ BU)

69. Minestrone
10 g olive oil or health-store vegetable fat
onion
50 g leek
celery leaves
50 g chard leaves
500 g vegetable broth (or water)
5 g lovage or thyme
¼ garlic clove
15 g rice
10 g butter

Sauté.
Cut small and cook slowly.
Add and cook for ½ hour.
Cook with the rest (15–20 min.).

Add to refine.
Season with: basil, parsley, chives
K = 153 E = 3 g F = 9 g CH = 14 g (= 1 BU)

70. Minestrone
5 g olive oil or health-food store
vegetable fat
onion, chopped
30 g leek stems, strips
30 g celery (celeriac), diced
30 g carrots, diced
50 g cabbage, strips
50 g potatoes, diced, mangold or
spinach leaves
100 g ripe tomatoes or
5 g tomato puree, diluted
500 g vegetable broth or water
15 g rice or soy pasta
10 g cheese, grated

Sauté briefly.
Add and cook thoroughly.
Briefly cook vegetables together.
Add and cook on low heat for 1 hour.
Cook together for 15 min.
Pour into soup bowl.
Season with: a pinch of salt, lovage, thyme
or other herbs.
K = 274 E = 8 g F = 13 g CH = 32 g
(= 2½ BU)

NB: The vegetables can BU arranged to suit the season and taste (e.g. cubes of young courgettes, yellow pumpkin instead of potatoes, tips of wild asparagus, green beans).

Vegetables

Cooked vegetables are subject to the same basic rules of nutrition and preparation as raw vegetables (i.e. cleanliness, freshness and careful preparation). Almost all vegetables can either be sautéed or cooked in a little vegetable broth. Where vegetables have to be parboiled in salted water, the water can be used for sauces or soups. Asparagus is an excep-

tion, since asparagus water is not beneficial to your health.
If fresh vegetables are hard to come by, frozen vegetables can be used (thaw as needed and then use immediately). It is important to use very little salt with all foods because of the danger of hypertension. Skilful use of herbs can easily replace salt.

71. Spinach, whole leaves, 1st option
Sort the spinach, remove thick stalks, wash thoroughly and drain.
5 g olive oil or health-food store vegetable fat
onion, chopped
½ garlic clove, chopped
250 g spinach, young
salt
nutmeg

Sauté until golden.
Add and cover and cook over low heat.
Season with: a little health-food store yeast extract.
K = 101 E = 7,5 g F = 5 g CH = 7 g (= ½ BU)
Adult winter spinach may have to be rinsed in salt water in order to remove its bitter taste.

72. Spinach, whole leaves, 2nd option*
250 g spinach
5 g butter, liquid
10 g cheese, grated

Prepare as above.
Sprinkle over the spinach.
K = 143 E = 10 g F = 8 g CH = 16 g (= 1½ BU)

73. Spinach, whole leaves, 3rd option
250 g spinach
5 g olive oil or health-food store vegetable fat
¼ onion, chopped
10 g pine seeds
Add water as needed.

Pour into pan, cover and cook over low heat.
Sauté to a golden colour, add spinach and continue to cook briefly.
K = 159 E = 8 g F = 10 g CH = 9 g (= 1 BU)

74. Spinach, chopped, 2nd option*
Prepare as described in "Whole leaves, first option"
250 g spinach
10 g olive oil or health-food store vegetable fat
¼ onion
15 g cream
50 g spinach, raw (opt.)

Place in pan, cover and cook over low heat until there is no more water, drain.
Then feed through the food processor or chop.
Sauté briefly and add the spinach, heat.
Add.
Mix or chop finely and add to the spinach.
Season with: peppermint leaves, sage, parsley (winter spinach may be blanched.)
K = 189 E = 10 g F = 12 g CH = 8 g (= ½ BU)

75. Lettuce
250 g lettuce
500 g water
10 g olive oil or health-food store vegetable fat
¼ onion
100 g vegetable broth
10 g cream

Halve, parboil until semi-soft, fold and place in baking dish.
Sauté until golden yellow and pour over the vegetables.
Add and cook in the oven for about 30–40 min.
Pour over 5 min before serving.
K = 155 E = 5 g F = 12 g CH = 5 g (= ½ BU)

76. Endive vegetables
250 g endive

Prepared like lettuce.
K = 131 E = 4 g F = 10 g CH = 5 g (= ½ BU)

77. Chicory
200 g chicory, prepared
5 g olive oil or health-food store vegetable fat and
50 g milk
50 g vegetable broth
very little salt
a few drops of lemon juice (opt.)
5 g butter

Cut a cross into the stalk.
Heat in a pan, then add chicory.
Add and cook over low heat for ½ hour.
Sprinkle over the prepared chicory.
K = 97 E = 3 g F = 7 g CH = 5 g (= ½ BU)

78. Chicory polonaise*
200 g chicory
1 egg, hard-boiled
5 g butter

Prepare as above.
Chop fine and pour over the prepared chicory.
To refine.

NB: instead of liquid butter, this can be refined with nut or almond puree.
Season with: onions, parsley, chives.
K = 143 E = 9 g F = 9 g CH = 5 g (= ½ BU)

79. Cabbage stems*
200 g cabbage stems, prepared
5 g olive oil or health-food store vegetable fat
30 g (= ¼) onion, chopped
50 g vegetable broth
a few drops of lemon juice
10 g cream, refined with egg yolk

Cut into 3 cm long pieces.
Sauté.

Add and cook until soft over low heat for ½ to ¾ hour.
Add.
K = 126 E = 8 g F = 5 g CH = 9 g (= 1 BU)

80. Cabbage stems or "false asparagus"
300 g cabbage stems, prepared
5 g olive oil or health-food store vegetable fat
¼ onion, chopped
30 g milk or a few drops of lemon juice
50 g vegetable broth

Cut into 10 cm long pieces.
Sauté, add.
Add and cook over low heat for ½ to ¾ hours until soft.

NB: the "asparagus" can also be served with grated cheese and 5 g liquid butter, or with curd sauce.
K = 137 E = 7 g F = 6 g CH = 10 g (= 1 BU)

81. Celery stalk
200 g celery sticks, prepared
5 g olive oil or health-food store vegetable fat
¼ onion, chopped
50 g vegetable broth
30 g milk or a little lemon juice

Cut into 8 cm long pieces.
Add and sauté everything.
Add and cook for ½ to ¾ hours until soft.
Add.
Season with: celery greens.
K = 101 E = 3 g F = 5 g CH = 9 g (= 1 BU)

82. Fennel
Trim tough parts, halve and rinse
1 large or 2 small fennels
5 g olive oil or health-food store vegetable fat
onion
50 g vegetable broth
30 g milk or a little lemon juice
 pinch of salt
10 g cream* or 10 g cheese*, grated

Halve fennel and place in pan.
Sauté and then pour over.
Add fennel and cook until soft.
Sprinkle grated cheese over the served fennel.
K = 189 E = 6 g F = 9 g CH = 20 g (= 1½ BU)

83. Cardoon
2 – 3 stems of cardoon
5 g olive oil or health-food store vegetable fat
lemon juice
100 g vegetable broth

Prepare and cut into 10 cm long pieces, place in pan.
Add liquid.
Cook everything for ¾ to 1 hour until soft.
Arrange on plate, sprinkle with 10 g cheese and add 5 g liquid butter.
Season with: lovage.
K = 193 E = 8 g F = 9 g CH = 18 g
(= 1½ BU)

84. Carrots, sautéed
5 g olive oil or health-food store vegetable fat
¼ onion, chopped
200 g carrots (sticks or julienne)
100 g vegetable broth

Sauté.
Add and cook for ½ to ¾ hours until soft.
Season with: parsley, marjoram or rosemary.
K = 119 E = 2 g F = 5 g CH = 16 g
(= 1½ BU)

85. Green beans
5 g olive oil or health-food store vegetable fat
¼ onion, chopped
garlic
250 g beans
savory
parsley
100 g vegetable broth
1 – 2 tomatoes, finely diced
pinch of salt

Sauté.
Add, cook about 1 hour.
K = 147 E = 8 g F = 5 g CH = 15 g
(= 1½ BU)

86. Dried beans (dried green beans)
30 g dried beans
(30 g dried beans = 265 g fresh beans)
Soak overnight, then drain.
Preparation like fresh green beans, reuse soak water, add mixed soybean flour to bind (opt.).
K = 147 E = 8 g F = 5 g CH = 15 g
(= 1½ BU)

87. Celery, sautéed
5 g olive oil or health-food store vegetable fat
¼ onion
200 g celery, prepared
5 g lemon juice or
10 g milk
100 g vegetable broth
15 g cream

Sauté.
Cut into small square slices and cook.
Add and cook for ½ to ¾ hours until soft.
Add to refine.
K = 182 E = 3 g F = 9 g CH = 19 g
(= 1½ BU)

88. Black salsify, sautéed
150 g black salsifies, prepared
5 g olive oil or health-food store vegetable fat
¼ onion
50 g milk or
5 g lemon juice
100 g vegetable broth
5 g cream

Cut into finger-length pieces and place in pan.
Sauté, add.
Pour over and cover and cook over low heat for 1 hour.
Add cream for refinement.
K = 200 E = 4 g F = 13 g CH = 27 g (= 2 BU)

89. Beetroot vegetables
Cut off the root tips and leaves to approx.
2 cm, wash thoroughly without damaging
the skin.
200 g beetroot
in lightly salted water
5 g olive oil or health-food store
vegetable fat
¼ onion, chopped
100 g vegetable broth
¼ laurel leaf
caraway
5 g soy flour, mixed cold
5 g cream
5 g lemon juice

Cook until soft, 2–3 hrs. (or in pressure
cooker about 25 min.). Peel, then cut into
fine slices.
Sauté, then add the vegetables.
Add, mix well and cook over low heat
for ¼ hour.
Add to the binding.
K = 154 E = 4 g F = 7 g CH = 17 g
(= 1½ BU)

90. Jerusalem artichoke
200 g Jerusalem artichoke
5 g olive oil or health-store vegetable fat
¼ onion, chopped
10 g cream

Cook like potatoes in the peel, then peel
and slice.
Sauté with Jerusalem artichoke.
Add cream to refine.
K = 211 E = 4 g F = 7 g CH = 32 g
(= 2½ BU)

91. Tomato vegetables
Pour boiling water over the tomatoes and
peel them (very ripe tomatoes can BU
peeled without boiling water).
5 g olive oil or health-food store
vegetable fat
10 g oil
¼ onion, chopped
250 g tomatoes
pinch of salt

garlic
5 g soy flour

Brown slightly in frying pan.
Cut into pieces, add to the onions and
sauté until slightly cooked.
Add and cook until done.
Use soy flour for binding.
Sprinkle the tomatoes with chopped
parsley, chives or other herbs.
Season with: rosemary, marjoram, basil,
laurel leaf.
K = 207 E = 4 g F = 15 g CH = 11 g (= 1 BU)

92. Tomatoes, baked
200 g tomatoes
5 g butter

Halve and place on greased tray or in
baking dish.
Put dabs of butter (or olive oil) on each
half and bake briefly in the oven.

NB: If desired, a tomato can be blended
(in blender or multi-blender) or chopped
very fine, then mixed with 5 g cream,
boiled briefly and poured over the prepared tomatoes.
Season with: parsley, onions (cooked with
the tomatoes).
K = 88 E = 2 g F = 6 g CH = 7 g (½ BU)

93. Tomatoes with cheese slices*
200 g tomatoes
30 g cheese

Prepare as above.
Cut cheese into thin slices the size of the
tomatoes and place on halved tomatoes.
Bake in the oven until the cheese melts.
K = 162 E = 10 g F = 10 g CH = 7 g (= ½ BU)

94. Tomatoes, stuffed
200 g tomatoes
15 g rice (5 g per tomato)
5 g butter
Herbs, vegetable broth (opt.)
Sprinkle with 10 g grated cheese* (opt.)
Cut off top and hollow out, chop tomato

flesh and mix with 5 g uncooked rice per tomato, season with herbs as desired, fill into hollowed tomatoes.
Put flakes of butter on top and cover with cut-off top.
Bake in the oven for 30 min at moderate heat.
Season with: onions, garlic, rosemary, thyme, basil, parsley, chives.
K = 172 E = 5 g F = 8 g CH = 18 g (= 1½ BU)

95. American tomatoes*
200 g nice tomatoes
1 egg, hard boiled
10 g mayonnaise
cold vegetable broth
gherkins, cress and radishes (opt.)

Cut tomatoes and egg into slices and alternate them on a plate like scales, salt lightly.
Dilute mayonnaise with cold vegetable broth and pour over the tomatoes.
Garnish with gherkins, cress and radishes (opt.).
K = 200 E = 8 g F = 15 g CH = 7 g (= ½ BU)

96. Tomatoes à la Provence
200 g tomatoes
pinch of salt
10 g cheese, grated
5 g cream or 15 g milk
20 g onion, chopped
10 g parsley

Halve tomatoes, salt, place on greased tray.
Mix and spread with a spoon on the tomatoes, bake briefly in the oven.
Mix and spread on the tomatoes.
K = 110 E = 6 g F = 6 g CH = 10 g (= 1 BU)

97. Tomatoes with scrambled eggs*
150 g tomatoes
pinch of salt
1 egg
5 g cream
5 g olive oil or health-food store vegetable fat

Halve and place on greased tray or in baking dish.
Whisk.
Melt in the omelette pan and stir the egg mixture over low heat until slightly flaky.
Immediately pour over the tomatoes.
K = 156 E = 7 g F = 10 g CH = 6 g (= ½ BU)

98. Courgettes, 1st option
The courgettes should be as young, tender, small and narrow as possible.
Wash well and cut off only the two ends.
5 g olive oil or health-food store vegetable fat
¼ onion, chopped
200 g courgettes
pinch of salt
rosemary, dill, parsley
5 g cream

Sauté courgettes.
Dice courgettes (remove the inner core if courgettes are full-grown).
Add and, if necessary, braise with vegetable broth until soft.
Add cream to refine.
K = 107 E = 3 g F = 6 g CH = 10 g (= 1 BU)

99. Courgettes, 2nd option
200 g courgettes
5 g olive oil
pinch of salt

Cut in half and place in flat pan.
Add to the mixture and braise in the oven or on the stove, covered over low heat (add vegetable broth if necessary).
Season with: rosemary, dill, parsley.
Serve with: tomato sauce, prepared as follows:
50 g tomatoes
pinch of salt
10 g cream*

Cut into pieces, cook briefly, season and strain.
Add cream to refine (or health-food store vegetable fat or 5 g fresh butter).

Tomato sauce, second option, prepared as follows:
5 g olive oil or health-food store vegetable fat
¼ onion
50 g tomatoes, peeled
pinch of salt
basil, rosemary or thyme

Sauté.
Dice
Add.
Cook together until soft.
K = 133 E = 2 g F = 11 g CH = 5 g (= ½ BU)

100. Bell peppers, green or yellow, sautéed
Preferable as a side dish.
200 g bell pepper
50 g onion
10 g olive oil

Cut into fine strips
Cook together in covered frying pan for ½ hour.
Season with: garlic, rosemary, basil, parsley.
K = 171 E = 3 g F = 11 g CH = 15 g (= 1½ BU)

101. Stuffed bell peppers*
200 g bell peppers
Salt lightly
5 g olive oil or health-food store vegetable fat
50 g onion, chopped
30 g rice
100 g tomatoes
5 g cheese, grated
5 g butter
100 g vegetable broth

Place in buttered baking dish.
See under "Tomato rice" (rice and tomatoes with 5 g health-food store vegetable fat, ¼ garlic clove, salt lightly, add 20 g vegetable broth, cook for about 15 – 20 min, add 5 g grated cheese).
Stuff the bell peppers.

Top up with vegetable broth, bake in the oven for ½ hour.
K = 276 E = 6 g F = 12 g CH = 34 g (= 3 BU)

NB: before preparation, briefly soak mature bell peppers in salted water, or leave them in cold water for 1 hour.

102. Peperonata
50 g bell peppers
50 g courgettes
50 g aubergines
50 g tomatoes
¼ onion
garlic
10 g olive oil
50 g potatoes

Halve, core and dice.
Peel and cut into larger dice.
Finely chop, steam.
Sauté the vegetables together.
Cut into 1 cm cubes, add and steam for 1 – 1½ hours. If too much juice is produced, heat uncovered until it reduces.
Season with: rosemary, thyme or basil, parsley.
K = 203 F = 4 g F = 10 g CH = 22 g (= 2 BU)

103. Aubergine
150 g aubergines, wash, peel
5 g olive oil or health-food store vegetable fat
¼ onion, chopped
salt
50 g vegetable broth
cooked tomato halves or tomato medley

Dice.
Sauté.
Add the aubergines and cook until soft.
Add.
Garnish.
K = 81 E = 2 g F = 5 g CH = 7 g (= ½ BU)

104. Aubergines*
200 g aubergines
10 g olive oil
50 g tomatoes

pinch of salt
20 g cheese, grated or sliced
5 g butter in flakes

Cut into slices.
Bake until soft, then pour into
casserole dish.
Cut into slices and place on top.
Sprinkle or lay over it.
Add and bake in the oven for ½ hour.
K = 280 E = 8 g F = 21 g CH = 13 g (= 1 BU)

105. Aubergines, stuffed
Prepare like the first aubergine recipe
200 g aubergines
(wash, peel)
10 g olive oil
100 g vegetable broth

Stuffing:
Rice stuffing (like stuffed bell peppers)
Cut into halves, hollow out slightly and
place in baking dish, with inner surface
facing up, coated with oil.
Fill up to half the aubergines and cover
and braise until semi-soft.
Fill in and finish baking covered.
K = 332 E = 6 g F = 18 g CH = 35 g (= 3 BU)

106. Artichokes
Cut off the stalks close to the artichokes.
Remove the lower hard leaves and cut off
the tips; halve and cut out the flower,
rinse with running water and rub the cut
surface with lemon juice.
150 g artichokes
500 g water and
5 g lemon juice
10 g mayonnaise (recipe no. 7* or 8)
or with
15 g vinaigrette (recipe no. 195)

Boil to soften the artichokes, about
¾ hour.
Then let them drain and arrange them on
a warm plate covered with napkin and
serve with mayonnaise or vinaigrette.
K = 92 E = 4 g F = – CH = 18 g (= 1½ BU)

107. Artichokes, sautéed
200 g artichokes
pinch of salt
15 g olive oil
50 g water

Cut out the tender, soft parts, wash and
rub with lemon, cut into thin slices.
Sprinkle.
Sauté until soft.
Continue cooking.
K = 261 E = 5 g F = 15 g CH = 24 g (= 2 BU)

108. Roman artichokes
200 g artichoke
(2 smaller ones or 1 large one)
pinch of salt
peppermint leaves, chopped
small clove of garlic
10 g olive oil
water

Peel the outermost leaves from top to
bottom until only the tender part remains,
cut off the tips, peel the stem to the pulp
and leave it 5 cm long. Thoroughly rub
with lemon and open the leaves slightly.
Sprinkle with salt, place peppermint and
garlic inside the artichokes. Cover the
bottom of the pan with oil, place the artichokes in the pan and braise with the pan
covered. Turn a few times, then fill up with
water to half the height of the artichokes
and cook until no water is left, then
continue to cook in oil for a short time.
K = 215 E = 5 g F = 10 g CH = 24 g (= 2 BU)

109. Asparagus
Wash the asparagus carefully so that it
does not break, then peel it.
300 g asparagus
500 g water
pinch of salt
10 g grated cheese* and
5 g butter
or
20 g sauce mayonnaise, recipe no. 7 or 8
or
20 g vinaigrette sauce, recipe no. 195

Cook in a large pan for 20–30 min until soft, remove with a slotted spoon and arrange on a plate covered with a napkin. Add the desired sauce ("melt").
K = 141 E = 8 g F = 8 g CH = 9 g (= 1 BU)

110. Corn on the cob
Use only corn cobs with tender and milky grains. Remove the green leaves and threads.
2 medium-sized corn cobs in approx.
½ l = 500 g water - salt water

Cook for 10–15 min until soft.
Arrange on a hot platter covered with a folded napkin. Serve with 10 g butter.
K = 184 E = 3 g F = 9 g CH = 19 g (= 1½ BU)

111. Cauliflower
200 g cauliflower
500 g water

Cut off leaves and stalk below the flower, peel stalk, keep tender leaves, soak in cold water for 1 hour, rinse well.
Cook for 20–30 min, then arrange on a warm, deep dish.
Season with: approx. 15–20 g butter sauce* with tarragon and lemon, or approx. 10 g butter, parsley, chives.
K = 134 E = 5 g F = 9 g CH = 8 g (= ½ BU)

112. Cauliflower polonaise
200 g cauliflower
½ egg, hard boiled
parsley
10 g grated cheese
5 g liquid (not brown) butter

Prepare as above.
Chop fine, mix cheese with parsley and sprinkle over the cauliflower.
Pour on butter.
K = 173 E = 11 g F = 13 g CH = 8 g (= ½ BU)

113. Broccoli (a kind of cauliflower)
Preparation like cauliflower
K = 173 E = 11 g F = 13 g CH = 8 g (= ½ BU)

114. Stachys
5 g olive oil or health-food store vegetable fat
20 g onion, chopped
200 g stachys
50 g vegetable broth
10 g cream or
5 g butter

Sauté.
Cook until soft.
For refining (like celery vegetables).
K = 224 E = 4 g F = 7 g CH = 34 g (= 3 BU)

115. Brussels sprouts, sautéed
5 g olive oil or health-food store vegetable fat
200 g Brussels sprouts, cleaned
500 g vegetable broth

Sauté briefly.
Add, cook together until soft for ½ hour.
When serving, pour on 15 g liquid butter* or olive oil.
Season with: Basil or thyme.

NB: If the Brussels sprouts are not tender, they can be briefly doused with hot water before cooking.
K = 154 E = 9 g F = 28 g CH = 14 g (= 1 BU)

116. Cabbage or white cabbage, sautéed
5 g olive oil or health-food store vegetable fat
¼ onion, chopped
250 g cabbage, young
50 g vegetable broth
Basil or lovage
(health-food store yeast extract, opt.), and nutmeg, caraway.

Sauté.
Cut into 2 cm wide strips.
Add, cook until the vegetables soften, pour vegetable broth and cook over low heat for ½ hour until soft.
Season.

NB: Green, mature cabbage must first be briefly doused in water.
K = 106 E = 3 g F = 5 g CH = 10 g (= 1 BU)

117. Cabbage, chopped
200 g cabbage
500 g water
5 g olive oil or health-food store vegetable fat
50 g onion, chopped
garlic
100 g vegetable broth
(or half milk, half vegetable broth)
10 g cream
Liq. phag or other yeast extract, nutmeg

Cut into pieces, cook until soft and drain, finely chop.
Sauté until golden.
Cook for ¼ an hour with the cabbage.
Add to refine.
Season with: caraway, parsley.
K = 142 E = 3 g F = 8 g CH = 11 g (= 1 BU)

118. Kale
Prepare like cabbage.
K = 142 E = 3 g F = 8 g CH = 11 g (= 1 BU)

119. Sour white cabbage
5 g olive oil or health-food store vegetable fat
with ¼ onion, chopped
250 g white cabbage, finely chopped or grated
5 g lemon juice and
50 g vegetable broth,
caraway seeds and salt

Sauté.
Sauté together.
Add and cook covered for 1 hour.
Season with: garlic, lovage, tomatoes, mushrooms.
K = 67 E = 4 g F = 1 g CH = 11 g (= 1 BU)

120. Sauerkraut
10 g olive oil or health-food store vegetable fat
¼ onion, chopped
250 g sauerkraut
25 g vegetable broth
30 g potatoes (raw)

Sauté briefly.
Add, separate gently with the fork and continue streaming briefly.
Add and cook on low heat for 1–2 hours, covered.
Grate in 10 min before serving.
K = 173 E = 4 g F = 10 g CH = 16 g (= 1½ BU)

121. Red cabbage
5 g olive oil or health-food store vegetable fat
¼ onion, chopped
250 g red cabbage, finely sliced
5–10 g rice and
lemon juice
100 g vegetable broth and
50 g grape juice or
apple juice
80 g apples, peeled, in slices
spread with 5 g butter
and simmer with 5 g liquid butter

Add and simmer together.
Deglaze and cook covered over a low flame for 1–1½ hours until soft.
Bake on a tray in the oven.
Gratinate.
K = 302 E = 5 g F = 14 g CH = 37 g (= 3 BU)

122. Kohlrabi, steamed
200 g kohlrabi
5 g olive oil or health-food store vegetable fat
¼ onion, chopped
100 g vegetable broth
pinch of salt
tender kohlrabi leaves, chopped
10 g cream

Cut into 4 pieces, then into fine slices.
Sauté and add the vegetables.
Add and cook covered for ½–1 hour.
Add last.

If you have no fresh, tender kohlrabi leaves, add chopped parsley.
Very tender kohlrabi can also only be cut into 4 pieces and cooked.
K = 135 E = 4 g F = 9 g CH = 10 g (= 1 BU)

123. Leek vegetables
200 g leek, prepared
5 g olive oil or health-food store vegetable fat
50 g vegetable broth
15 g cream
10 g grated cheese* (opt.)

Cut into 10 cm long pieces, layer in the frying pan.
Add, cover and roast slowly.
Add last.
K = 197 E = 8 g F = 12 g CH = 13 g (= 1 BU)

124. Onion vegetables
5 g olive oil or health-food store vegetable fat
150 g pearl onions
50 g vegetable broth

Sauté slowly.
Add and cook for another ¾ hours.
K = 112 E = 2 g F = 5 g CH = 14 g (= 1 BU)

125. White beans with tomatoes
50 g beans, white
150 g vegetable broth
pinch of salt
5 g olive oil or health-food store vegetable fat
¼ onion, chopped
100 g tomatoes
½ garlic clove

Soak overnight and drain.
Boil the beans until soft.
Sauté.
Peel and cut into cubes, cook together.
Add everything to the boiled beans, continue to cook for a few min.
K = 237 E = 12 g F = 5 g CH = 33 g (= 3 BU)

126. Mixed vegetables
5 g olive oil or health-food store vegetable fat
¼ onion, chopped
50 g celery
50 g carrots
100 g vegetable broth
50 g cauliflower
50 g peas or beans
100 g vegetable broth
100 g spinach
5 g health-food store vegetable fat
20 g onion, chopped

Sauté.
Dice finely and sauté.
Add and sauté until fully cooked.
Boil in a little milk water until soft.
Sauté together until soft.
Cut into small pieces and cook together
Then mix with the cooked vegetables or arrange them in layers.
Melt 5 g butter over it.

NB: Other vegetables can also be used for this dish.
K = 266 E = 9 g F = 15 g CH = 21 g (= 2 BU)

127. Stuffing for "stuffed vegetables"*
Rice stuffing:
30 g rice
60 g vegetable broth
1 egg
15 g cheese, grated
Herbs, chopped
20 g mushrooms, chopped

Cook until soft.
Mix all ingredients with the cooked rice.
K = 236 E = 12 g F = 11 g CH = 22 g (= 2 BU)

Salads of cooked vegetables

Carrots, celery (celeriac), beetroot, green beans, cauliflower and stachys are particularly suitable for these salads.
The vegetables are cooked in vegetable

broth or water and then finely chopped (cubes, slices, florets).
Prepared with salad dressing, recipe no. 6 or with
mayonnaise, recipe no. 7 or 8, diluted.
Cauliflower can also be coated with mayonnaise, recipe 7 or 8. Season with onions and chopped herbs.

128. Potato salad, 1st option
200 g potatoes in the peel
50 g vegetable broth, hot
15 g olive oil with
15 g lemon juice
5 g cream and
5 g onion, chopped

Cook, then peel and slice.
Add and let rest briefly.
Whisk well and mix with the potatoes.
Season with: Borage, chives, parsley, lemon balm, marjoram, thyme, dill
K = 328 E = 4 g F = 17 g CH = 40 g (= 3½ BU)

129a. Potato salad, 2nd option
200 g potatoes (in the skin)
100 g vegetable broth
15 g lemon juice
5 g onion, chopped
pinch of salt, nutmeg
14 g mayonnaise, recipe no. 7* or 8

Cook, then peel the cooked, still hot potatoes and slice.
Add and let rest briefly.
Mix with the potatoes.
K = 271 E = 4 g F = 11 g CH = 39 g (= 3 BU)

130. Potato salad with cucumbers
200 g potatoes
50 g cucumber
10 g olive oil
10 g lemon juice

Prepare as above (potato salad, 1st option)
Grate on a coarse grater.
Add and mix with potato salad.

Season with: dill or borage, chives, parsley, finely chopped onion. Rub bowl with garlic.
K = 428 E = 4 g F = 37 g CH = 41 g (= 3½ BU)

131. Salad Niçoise*
80 g potatoes, peeled, cooked
80 g tomatoes
10 g radish
1 egg, hard boiled
20 g cucumber
15 g olive oil
15 g lemon juice
lettuce leaves

Cut into slices.
Prepare salad dressing and mix with the vegetables and egg.
Mix with the salad briefly before serving.
Season with: parsley, chives or dill, lemon balm, borage.
K = 301 E = 9 g F = 20 g CH = 20 g (= 1½ BU)

132. Rice salad
30 g rice
150 g water
15 g oil
10 g lemon juice
10 g onion, chopped
50 g tomatoes, finely diced

Cook the rice, rinse briefly and let cool.
Whisk sauce, mix with rice.
Mix lightly.
Season with: chives, parsley or basil.
Arrange the finished salad on lettuce leaves and serve in bowls for festive occasions.
K = 247 E = 2 g F = 16 g CH = 23 g (= 2 BU).

133. Russian salad*
50 g carrots
50 g celery (celeriac)
50 g peas
50 g potatoes in the jacket
15 g lemon juice
pinch of salt
15 g mayonnaise, recipe no. 7

Cook each vegetable separately until soft in vegetable broth or salt water, let cool.
Dice carrots, celery and potatoes.
Mix with the cooled vegetables.
Mix thoroughly.
Garnish with gherkins, tomatoes and cress.
K = 378 E = 12 g F = 16 g CH = 45 g (= 4 BU)

134. Celery salad with mayonnaise*
150 g celery (celeriac), raw
10 g lemon juice
10 g walnuts, coarsely chopped
15 g mayonnaise and
10 g cream

Cut into match-sized strips, grate if necessary.
Mix in mayonnaise.
K = 255 E = 4 g F = 19 g CH = 14 g (= 1 BU)

135. Russian eggs*
1 egg, hard boiled
15 g mayonnaise, recipe no. 7
pinch of salt
health-food store yeast extract

Peel, halve and remove the egg yolk, strain through fine-meshed sieve.
Mix with the egg yolk and inject with the piping bag into the hollowed-out eggs.

NB: Use the eggs to garnish salad platters for special occasions. Mix part of the mixture with finely chopped herbs or tomato puree (opt.).
K = 207 E = 6 g F = 20 g CH = 1 g (= 0 BU)

136. Vegetable brawn
200 g vegetable broth, lukewarm
3–4 g agar-agar[1], powdered
a few drops of lemon juice
health-food store yeast extract
pinch of salt

1 egg, sliced
50 g tomatoes, diced
gherkins, pickled gherkins
50 g cauliflower florets, cooked
30 g peas, cooked
30 g beans, cooked

Dissolve the agar-agar in vegetable broth and boil.
For seasoning.
Place a little brawn in a rinsed mould and let harden.
Garnish with egg and vegetable slices, then pour vegetable broth over it again, let harden, repeat until the moulds are filled.
Turn over the cooled brawns and use to garnish salad platters.
K = 151 E = 11 g F = 6 g CH = 10 g (= 1 BU)

Sandwiches

Sandwiches are popular as a starter and for summer dinners, and to take along on hikes and journeys.
Different spreads and ingredients can be combined in new ways every time. The more attractive and fresher the sandwiches look, the more appetising they are.
For diabetics, bread must be thinly sliced and only wholemeal bread used. The bread should be at least one day old so that it can be cut into thin slices.
The calculation of the bread units was based on 2 slices = 40 g bread.
Wheat wholemeal bread:
100 g: K = 202 = EW = 7.1g F = 0.9g CH = 41.4g = (3.5 BE)
Only wholemeal breads should be used.

137. Basic spreads
30 g lean quark
5 g butter

Stir until fluffy.
K = 163 E = 8 g F = 5 g CH = 20 g (= 2 BU)

---
1 Agar-agar is plant-based jelly powder used for vegetable and fruit spreads, sauces and puddings etc. instead of animal gelatine.

or
40 g cream quark*
health-food store yeast extract
and chives, herbs
caraway or tomato puree

Mix in.
K = 135 E = 10 g F = 1 g CH = 21 g (= 2 BU)

or
10 g herb butter* with
dill or borage
with a little lemon juice
or milk

Mix.
K = 173 E = 3 g F = 9 g CH = 19 g
(= 1½ BU)

or
10 g cheese spread*
5 g cream

Strain through a sieve and stir until fluffy.
K = 150 g E = 6 g F = 5 g CH = 19 g
(= 1½ BU)

or
30 g Emmental cheese* or
Gruyère cheese*
20 g milk and possibly some caraway seeds

Grate finely, mix
Leave for ½ hour.
K = 234 E = 12 g E = 11 g CH = 21 g
(= 2 BU)
Nut and almond puree are also suitable for spreading on bread.

Garnishes:
The bread with spread can BU garnished as follows:
with raw carrots or celery (celeriac).
with tomato (sliced, diced, etc.), fresh cucumber, radish, cress, onion (rings), walnuts, parsley, chives etc.
with chopped egg*, mixed with mayonnaise*.

Cress with chopped egg* and some mayonnaise* or salad dressing.
Asparagus tips with mayonnaise* etc.

Potato dishes

138. Potatoes in jacket
yellow or red potatoes are particularly suitable.
120 g potatoes
water, lightly salted

Brush and wash.
Place in a pan with perforated insert or wire sieve, add water to the insert. Add the potatoes, cover and cook for 30–40 min or in a pressure cooker according to instructions.
K = 95 E = 2 g F = 0 g CH = 20 g (= 1½ BU)

139. Baked potatoes
120 g potatoes
5 g olive oil

Brush, wash.
Score the skin on upper side three or four times, brush with oil and bake for 30–40 min on greased sheet at medium heat.
K = 141 E = 2 g F = 5 g CH = 20 g (= 1½ BU)

140. Quark potatoes
120 g potatoes
5 g olive oil
Stuffing:
50 g lean quark
10 g milk
chives or caraway seeds
or marjoram

Prepare as above, cut a groove into the top of the potatoes and prepare them as baked potatoes.
Stir until fluffy and mix with the other ingredients.
Use a piping bag to apply on the groove of the baked potatoes (can also be served with baked potatoes).
K = 205 E = 12 g F = 6 g CH = 23 g (= 2 BU)

141. Caraway or sesame seed potatoes
120 g potatoes, narrow, long shape
10 g olive oil
10 g caraway seeds lightly salted

Brush off, wash and halve through the narrow middle.
Mix and dab onto the cut surface of the potatoes, place on greased tray with cut surface facing down, brush with oil and bake at medium heat for ¾ hour.
K = 195 E = 2 g F = 10 g CH = 23 g (= 2 BU)

142. Bouillon potatoes
120 g potatoes
100 g vegetable broth
10 g butter

Wash, peel, halve or cut in pieces and cook in vegetable broth until soft.
Sprinkle over potatoes.
Season with: lovage, onion skin, thyme, laurel leaf.
K = 187 E = 2 g F = 9 g CH = 23 g (= 2 BU)

143. Parsley potatoes
120 g peeled potatoes
water
10 g fresh butter
5 g parsley, chopped

Cut lengthwise in four pieces.
Steam potatoes in sieve.
Melt, add parsley.
Mix with potatoes and serve.
K = 179 E = 2 g F = 8 g CH = 23 g (= 2 BU)

144. Cream potatoes
120 g peeled potatoes
5 g olive oil or health-food store vegetable fat
100 g vegetable broth
5 g cream, milk (opt.)
parsley

Slice, briefly steam potatoes and cook until soft with vegetable broth.
Add last.
Sprinkle on.
Season with: thyme, small cloves, nutmeg, health-store yeast extract, onion golden yellow roast.
K = 162 E = 3 g F = 7 g CH = 23 g (= 2 BU)

145. Potatoes with tomatoes
5 g olive oil or health-store vegetable fat
½ small onion
120 g potatoes
100 g vegetable broth
1 small tomato
10 g cream

Roast the onion to a light brown, add the peeled, sliced potatoes and cook until semi-soft in vegetable broth.
Peel, slice, add and finish cooking.
Add last.
Season with: marjoram or rosemary or thyme, nutmeg (opt.).
K = 144 E = 1 g F = 3 g CH = 25 g (= 2 BU)

146. Potato puree
120 g potatoes
100 g water, lightly salted
20 g butter*, melted or olive oil

Wash, peel and cut in pieces.
Steam until soft.
Add.
Season with: finely chopped sun-dried tomatoes, golden sautéed onion (rings).
Squirt onto warm platter directly through the potato press.
K = 256 E = 2 g F = 17 g CH = 23 g (= 2 BU)

147. Mashed potato
180 g potatoes
water
5 g butter
50 g milk
nutmeg

Peel, chop in pieces, steam until soft, strain through potato press.
Heat butter and milk, add potatoes, stir

until fluffy and season. Arrange on a hot plate, dip a knife in hot water and garnish with puree.
K = 225 E = 5 g F = 6 g CH = 37 g
(= 3 BU)

148. Potato dumplings
180 g potatoes
50 g milk
10 g butter* or olive oil

Prepare like mashed potatoes.
Dip a small ladle in liquid butter, cut out the ploughs and arrange on a hot pan.
Season with: nutmeg.
K = 263 E = 5 g F = 10 g CH = 37 g
(= 3 BU)

149. Potato cakes
180 g peeled potatoes
1 yolk
5 g soy flour
5 g olive oil or health-food store vegetable fat or

Steam until soft and strain.
Mix all ingredients.
Form cakes and bake on both sides.
Season with: nutmeg, marjoram, basil.
K = 277 E = 8 g F = 11 g CH = 35 g
(= 3 BU)

150. Roast potatoes
120 g peeled potatoes
100 g vegetable broth
5 g olive oil or health-food store vegetable fat
10 g cream* or olive oil

Halve, place in baking dish with the cut side facing down.
Add sauce and roast in the oven until the vegetable broth has thickened.
Turn over and roast until the cut surfaces are slightly browned.
Prepare roast potatoes with the cut facing up and sprinkle with chopped parsley.
K = 174 E = 3 g F = 8 g CH = 23 g
(= 2 BU)

151. Princess potatoes*
120 g potatoes
water
salt
10 g cheese, grated
1 egg
100 g milk
nutmeg and salt
5 g butter

Steam, peel and cut into thick slices, place in baking dish.
Whisk the ingredients and pour over.
Place the butter in pieces on the potatoes and bake in the oven for 10 to 15 min.
K = 248 E = 8 g F = 11 g CH = 28 g
(= 2 BU)

152. Potato pancakes
180 g potatoes
10 g olive oil or health-food store vegetable fat
Potatoes, lightly salted

Cook one day before use, then peel and slice thinly or grate with a coarse grater.
Heat in the frying pan.
Place in a frying pan, cover the potatoes and cook over medium heat until brown, then cover and finish cooking the potatoes, turning them several times.
Form cakes, let a light brown crust form at the bottom and turn it over onto the plate.

NB: If desired, sauté chopped onions in butter before adding the potatoes to the pan.
K = 233 E = 4 g F = 9 g CH = 34 g
(= 3 BU)

153. Lyon potatoes
5 g olive oil or health-food store vegetable fat
10 g olive oil
120 g peeled potatoes
salt
50 g onion, cut into strips

Heat up.

Slice and bake in hot fat until semi-soft.
Sprinkle on.
Add the onions and finish baking.
K = 257 E = 3 g F = 15 g CH = 28 g
(= 2 BU)

154. Potato wedges (cooked raw)
120 g potatoes
5 g olive oil or health-food store vegetable fat
10 g olive oil

Peel and cut into wedges, dry in a cloth.
Heat and add the potatoes, cook covered for a short time, add a little salt and continue cooking covered for about ½ hour.
K = 235 E = 2 g F = 14 g CH = 23 g (= 2 BU)

155. "Schlosskartoffel" potatoes
180 g potatoes
salt
water
5 g olive oil or health-food store vegetable fat

Quarter lengthwise and round off the edges.
Steam until semi-soft.
Heat, add the potatoes and bake them slowly in the oven or on the stove, turning carefully a few times until the potatoes are golden yellow.
K = 193 E = 4 g F = 5 g CH = 34 g (= 3 BU)

156. Potato slices with spinach
120 g peeled potatoes
100 g vegetable broth
100 g spinach
10 g cheese*, grated
5 g butter

Cut lengthwise into 1 cm thick slices.
Cook the potatoes carefully until soft and place them on a buttered tray.
Prepare as leaf spinach, recipe no. 71, and add to potatoes.
Sprinkle over.
Add in small pieces and bake briefly in the oven.

K = 215 E = 8 g F = 9 g CH = 26 g (= 2 BU)

157. Potatoes with kale (stew)
5 g olive oil or health-store vegetable fat
½ small onion, chopped
100 g kale, finely chopped
120 g potatoes, diced
200 g vegetable broth
5 g butter

Steam.
Steam together.
Add and cook for ½ to ¾ hours.
Sprinkle over the potatoes.
Season with: finely chopped caraway, marjoram, nutmeg (basil).
K = 212 E = 4 g F = 11 g CH = 25 g (= 2 BU)

CEREAL DISHES

Rice dishes

For all rice dishes we use whole-grain rice with silver skin (e.g. in Switzerland Ostigliato rice or Demeter whole-grain rice)

158. Japanese rice
10 g olive oil or health-food store vegetable fat
40 g rice
100 g vegetable broth
5 g butter flakes

Steam the rice, add bouillon with onion (1 small laurel leaf, 1 clove) and cook for 15 min.
Rice should be grainy; let cool.
Heat, add the rice and fry until hot.
Add to finished rice.
K = 248 E = 2 g F = 14 g CH = 26 (= 2 BU)

159. Risotto*
3 g olive oil or health-store vegetable fat
½ small onion, chopped
40 g rice
100 g to 150 g vegetable broth
or water

3 g fresh butter
10 g grated cheese

Steam rice with onion.
Add hot and cook for 15 min.
Finally mix with a fork.
K = 239 E = 5 g F = 10 g CH = 27 g
(= 2½ BU)

160. Saffron rice*
Prepare like risotto, dissolve a pinch of saffron powder in bouillon and add to the rice.
Season with: dried mushrooms, finely chopped, fresh herbs to taste, rosemary.
K = 239 E = 5 g F = 10 g CH = 27 g
(= 2½ BU)

161. Riz Creol
5 g olive oil or health-food store vegetable fat
½ small onion, chopped
40 g rice
100 g water or vegetable broth

Sauté until the rice is glossy.
Add hot and cook for 15 to 20 min.
Season with: laurel, clove.
K = 171 E = 2 g F = 6 g CH = 26 g
(= 2 BU)

162. Riz Créol with vegetables
5 g olive oil or health-food store vegetable fat
10 g vegetables, finely diced
(leek, celery, carrots).
40 g rice
100 g vegetable broth

Steam everything together.
Add hot and cook for 15–20 min.
Season with: laurel leaf, clove, freshly chopped herbs (opt.).
K = 175 E = 2 g F = 6 g CH = 27 g
(= 2 BU)

163. Tomato rice
5 g olive oil or health-store vegetable fat
½ small onion, chopped
garlic
40 g rice
100 g tomatoes
100 g vegetable broth
5 g fresh butter
10 g grated cheese*

Sauté.
Sauté together until glossy.
Peel and dice, add.
Add and cook for 15–20 min.
Mix in last.
K = 270 E = 4 g F = 13 g CH = 30 g
(= 2½ BU)

164. Risotto with bel peppers*
5 g olive oil
10 g onion, chopped
½ bell pepper, cut into strips
40 g rice
80 g vegetable broth
10 g cheese, grated

Sauté.
Sauté together.
Add and cook for 15 min in the oven or on the stove until soft.
Mix in last.
If the bell pepper is too hot, the thick parts can be cut and placed in cold water for 1 hour before cooking.
K = 235 E = 6 g F = 13 g CH = 23 g (= 2 BU)

165. Rice with courgettes
5 g olive oil or health-food store vegetable fat
10 g onion, chopped
100 g tender courgettes
vegetable broth
or water
40 g rice
100 g water or vegetable broth
5 g fresh butter

Steam.
Dice and cook for 10 min.
Add in, then add the rice and gradually add liquid until a risotto is formed.

K = 224 E = 3 g F = 10 g CH = 29 g
(= 2½ BU)

166. Rice with peas
5 g olive oil or health-food store vegetable fat
onion, chopped
40 g peas, shelled
50 g vegetable broth
5 g health-food store vegetable fat
40 g rice
100 g water
5 g fresh butter
(grated cheese, opt.)

Steam.
Add and steam lightly, then cook until soft.
Prepare the risotto.
Add the cooked peas.
Put over the rice prepared for serving.
Season with: parsley, chopped, possibly cloves.
K = 301 E = 7 g F = 13 g CH = 31 g
(= 2½ BU)

167. Rice with spinach
5 g olive oil or health-food store vegetable fat
onion, chopped
100 g spinach, coarsely chopped
40 g rice
100 g vegetable broth or water (hot)
5 g fresh butter

Sauté.
Sauté together.
Add and cook for 15–20 min.
Mix in last.
Season with: nutmeg and peppermint.
K = 234 E = 5 g F = 10 g CH = 29 g
(= 2½ BU)

168. Rice gratin with tomatoes*
5 g olive oil or health-food store vegetable fat
onion, chopped
40 g rice
100 g vegetable broth
100 g tomatoes, sliced
5 g fresh butter
10 g cheese, grated

Steam.
Add and steam all together.
Add hot and boil for 15–20 min.
Place tomato slices and rice in layers in a buttered baking dish.
Add the dabs and bake in the oven for 10 min.
Sprinkle with cheese.
K = 292 E = 6 g F = 13 g CH = 31 g
(= 2½ BU)

169. Rice ring or rice head
40 g Japanese rice, Riz Créol, risotto or saffron rice can be placed in a ring form, pudding mould or cups rinsed with cold water and turned onto a plate.
Rice ring filled with tomato vegetables.
Rice head with 100 g white mushrooms, garnished with tomatoes and slices of an egg.
Rice heads garnished with braised, half tomatoes.
K = 290 E = 6 g F = 13 g CH = 31 g
(= 2½ BU)

Other cereal dishes

170. Maize porridge
40 g maize
20 g soy semolina
250 g water
100 g milk
salt
5 g fresh butter

Boil milk and lightly salted water, stir in maize and soy semolina, boil while stirring constantly, continue boiling for an hour and stir often.
Place butter dabs on the prepared porridge.
K = 301 E = 15 g F = 9 g CH = 39 g (= 3 BU)

171. Polenta
30 g olive oil
250 g water
40 g maize
nutmeg
5 g fresh butter
10 g grated cheese*

Grease the pan with oil, add water, bring to boil, stir in corn.
Add then cook for 5 min over low heat, stirring constantly, then cook for about 1 hour over low heat (or in cooking box).
K = 508 E = 6 g F = 39 g CH = 29 g
(= 2½ BU)

172. Maize slices*
50 g maize
20 g soy semolina
250 g milk
salt
1 egg, scrambled

Prepare like maize porridge, then spread on board and let cool. Slice, coat with egg mixture.
Place the unfried maize slices on a well-greased baking tray, bake lightly in a hot oven, then
place 30 g sliced cheese on maize slices and bake until cheese melts.
K = 618 E = 32 g F = 29 g CH = 50 g
(= 4 BU)

173. Hirsotto with vegetables
5 g olive oil or health-food store vegetable fat
10 g onion, chopped
100 g diced vegetables
(leek, celery, carrots).
30 g millet
100 g vegetable broth
10 g cheese, grated*
5 g fresh butter

Steam all together.
Add and cook for 20 min.
Add when serving.
K = 285 E = 7 g F = 14 g CH = 30 g
(= 2½ BU)

174. Hirsotto
3 g olive oil or health-food store vegetable fat
½ small onion, chopped
40 g millet
150 g vegetable broth, hot
10 g grated cheese*
5 g fresh butter, in flakes

Sauté until glossy.
Add and cook for 20 min.
Add when serving.
K = 256 E = 7 g F = 13 g CH = 26 g (= 2 BU)

175. Buckwheat groats
40 g buckwheat
100 g water
salt
10 g fresh butter or
nut or almond puree
50 g cold milk (cream, opt.)
fruit concentrate (opt.)

Soak for 24 hours.
Cook in covered pan for 1 hour or steam in a pressure cooker until soft.
Mix in last.
Serve together.
K = 256 E = 5 g F = 11 g CH = 33 g (= 3 BU)

176. Buckwheat meal
40 g buckwheat
100 g water
salt
20 g cream* or olive oil, fruit concentrate (opt.)

Soak for 24 hours, strain the soaked grains, chop or mix and cook in the soaking water for ½ hour.
Serve together.
K = 195 E = 5 g F = 5 g CH = 31 g
(= 2½ BU)

177. Roasted oat flakes*
3 g olive oil or health-food store vegetable fat
10 g onion, chopped
20 g oat flakes
20 g soy flakes
100 g leek, celery (celeriac) or spinach
100 g vegetable broth or milk
1 egg, scrambled in
10 g milk
10 g health-food store vegetable fat

Steam everything together.
Add, cook to a thick paste, then spread on board and let cool, cut into rectangles.
Place the rectangles in it.
Heat and bake the roasted oat flakes to a golden yellow on both sides.
K = 434 E = 20 g F = 24 g CH = 30 g
(= 2½ BU)

178. Omelettes, French*
2 eggs
15 g milk
salt, nutmeg
5 g fresh butter

Whisk all ingredients thoroughly; separate egg whites and beat them, then fold into mixture (opt.).
Heat in omelette pan, add the egg mixture and stir lightly with a fork. Fold when the mixture is semi-firm, finish cooking it and place it on a warm plate while the omelette is still moist.
K = 193 E = 12 g F = 15 g CH = 1 g
(= 0 BU)

179. Herbal omelettes*
Ingredients and preparation as above.
10 g herbs, chopped
(chives, parsley etc.)

Add, then prepare in omelette pan
Finish as above.
K = 199 E = 12 g F = 15 g CH = 2 g (= 0 BU)

180. Omelettes, French, with tomatoes*
Ingredients and preparation as above.

100 g tomatoes
5 g olive oil or health-food store vegetable fat
20 g onion, chopped

Peel and dice.
Steam, add tomatoes and steam until the juice is cooked.
Cut the omelette in the middle and add the tomatoes.
K = 261 E = 13 g F = 20 g CH = 6 g
(= ½ BU)

181. Soy omelettes
20 g soy flour
20 g flour
50 g milk
salt
5 g olive oil
5 g butter

Mix everything well, then let stand for one hour.
Mix into the dough.
Place in pan and bake lightly.
K = 274 E = 11 g F = 15 g CH = 20 g
(= 1½ BU)

182. Spinach pudding*
3 g olive oil or health-food store vegetable fat
1 small onion, chopped
1 garlic clove
150 g spinach, raw, chopped
20 g wholemeal bread in
30 g vegetable broth or milk
salt
1 yolk, beat egg whites
nutmeg, lovage
10 g grated cheese

Sauté.
Sauté together.
Soak, chop.
Mix ingredients well, then fold in the beaten egg whites.
Place the finished mixture in buttered dish sprinkled with wholemeal bread-

crumbs, cook in water bath (for a longer time in oven, opt.).
K = 313 E = 18 g F = 17 g CH = 20 g (= 1½ BU)

183. Cheese sandwiches*
30 g (1 slice) wholemeal bread
50 g milk
3 g olive oil or health-food store vegetable fat
15 g soy flour
30 g grated cheese

Turn slices in milk and place on greased tray.
Prepare Béchamel sauce, recipe no. 185.
Mix with the cooled sauce and spread over the bread slices.
Bake in a hot oven for about 10 min.
K = 317 E = 17 g F = 17 g CH = 22 g (= 2 BU)

184. Cheese casserole*
5 g butter
20 g soy flour
100 g milk
salt, nutmeg
1 yolk, scrambled and
30 g grated cheese
1 egg white
Béchamel sauce, recipe no. 185

Mix with the sauce.
Beat the egg and fold it in last, pour everything into the buttered casserole dish, cover and precook for 20–30 min in water bath, bake in oven for 20 min (water bath), medium heat.
K = 389 E = 23 g F = 26 g CH = 11 g (= 1 BU)

Sauces
Sauces should be used sparingly.

185. Béchamel sauce
10 g olive oil or health-food store vegetable fat
or butter
10 g soy flour

50 g milk
50 g vegetable broth

Warm.
Stir in and cook briefly.
Add the liquid slowly, stirring constantly, and cook for 10 min.
Season with: nutmeg
K = 153 E = 5 g F = 12 g CH = 5 g (= ½ BU)

186. Herbal sauce
Prepare Béchamel sauce
10 g fresh chopped herbs such as parsley, lovage, chervil, basil, tarragon etc.

Like recipe no. 185
Add.
K = 218 E = 8 g F = 17 g CH = 6 g (= ½ BU)

187. Tomato sauce, 1st option
5 g olive oil or health-food store vegetable fat
10 g onion, chopped
garlic
50 g carrots, celery, leek
100 g tomatoes
15 g soy flour
100 g vegetable broth or water
5 g liquid butter

Steam lightly.
Cut the vegetables coarsely and steam together.
Cut in pieces and cook together until juice disappears.
Sprinkle
Add, cook for about 10 min and strain.
Add last to refine.
Season with: laurel leaf, rosemary, thyme.
K = 190 E = 6 g F = 16 g CH = 8 g (= ½ BU)

188. Tomato sauce, 2nd option
150 g tomatoes
5 g cream (or fresh butter)

Cut in pieces, steam until soft and strain.
Add last to refine.
Season with: chives, basil, rosemary.
K = 41 E = 2 g F = 2 g CH = 6 g (= ½ BU)

189. Onion sauce
5 g olive oil or health-store vegetable fat
50 g onions, cut into strips
15 g soy flour
100 g vegetable broth
3 g fresh butter

Steam until golden yellow.
Add and cook for 20 min. If necessary, strain the finished sauce.
Add last to refine.
Season with: nutmeg, basil.
K = 151 E = 6 g F = 10 g CH = 7 g (= ½ BU)

190. Horseradish sauce
Prepare Béchamel sauce, recipe no. 185
10 g horseradish

Add to the finished sauce finely grated and boil for another 5 min, stirring constantly.
K = 161 E = 5 g F = 12 g CH = 6 g (= ½ BU)

191. White mushroom sauce, for refinement
5 g olive oil or health-food store vegetable fat
½ small onion, chopped
60 g white mushrooms
15 g soy flour
200 g vegetable broth
salt
5 g lemon juice
15 g cream

Stew briefly.
Cut into fine slices and steam for ¼ hour.
Sprinkle.
Add and cook for about 10 min.
Add last to refine.
K = 170 E = 7 g F = 12 g CH = 6 g (= ½ BU)

192. Bell pepper sauce
5 g olive oil or health-food store vegetable fat
10 g onion, chopped
20 g bell pepper, cut into fine strips
15 g soy flour
100 g vegetable broth
15 g cream* or olive oil

Steam everything slightly together.
Sprinkle.
Add and cook for 20 min.
Add at the end to refine.
Season with: laurel leaf.
K = 158 E = 6 g F = 11 g CH = 6 g (= ½ BU)

193. Mayonnaise sauce* (for 4 persons)
15 g yolk
2 g lemon juice
150 g olive oil
salt
health-food store yeast extract (opt.)

Mix the egg well with a few drops of lemon juice. Add the oil drop by drop while stirring with whisk.
If the mayonnaise grows too thick, dilute with a little lemon juice. Season to taste.
K = 1440 E = 2 g F = 154 g CH = 0 g (= 0 BU)

194. Mayonnaise made with soy instead of egg (for 4 persons)
8 g soy flour
30 g water
100 g olive oil
20 g lemon juice

Mix to a smooth consistency.
Add alternatingly, stirring constantly with whisk.
Season with: yeast extract and onions, chopped, and herbs.
K = 982 E = 4 g F = 101 g CH = 6 g (= ½ BU)

195. Vinaigrette (for 2 persons)
15 g olive oil
15 g peanut oil
25 g lemon juice
10 g water or vegetable broth
50 g onion, chopped
1 egg, hard boiled, chopped
20 g gherkins, finely chopped

parsley or chives
salt
20 g diced tomatoes

Mix all ingredients well with whisk.
As garnish.
K = 378 E = 7 g F = 35 g CH = 7 g (= ½ BU)

Desserts

These recipes are for one person. Sorbose and laevulose are preferred for sweetening, since they do not need insulin to be processed in the metabolism. Nevertheless, the volumes must be determined with care, since these substances may also cause glycation of the inner layer of the vessels if reading the blood at high concentrations, which consequently may cause hypertension and arteriosclerosis.

196. Strawberries in lemon juice
150 g strawberries, prepared
25 g lemon (juice)
15 g laevoral or
sorbitol (Sionon)

Halve large strawberries, sweeten and pour lemon juice over them.
K = 132 E = 1 g F = 0 g CH = 30 g (= 2½ BU)

197. Fruit salad
10 g laevoral or sorbitol in
50 g water
50 g orange juice
(or pure apple juice)
8 g lemon juice
150 g apricots, peaches, melons, apples, pears (soft variety) or red cherries (pitted), or any kind of berry

Boil and then let cool.
Add.
Select and compose according to the season.
Finely slice the fruit and add to syrup.
Garnish with contrasting fruits berries (opt.).

K = 148 E = 2 g F = 0 g CH = 34 g (= 3 BU)

198. Fruit jelly
100 g fruit juice
20 g laevoral or sorbitol
3 g agar-agar[1] powder
(or 1 g pectin)
5 g whipped cream (opt.)

Whisk well and heat on low heat until the agar-agar has completely dissolved, then mix well with the agar-agar and immediately arrange in glasses or bowls.
As garnish.
K = 158 E = 1 g F = 1 g CH = 33 g (= 3 BU)

199. Apple mash
150 g apples
10 g laevoral or sorbitol
cinnamon or lemon peel (grated) for refining
25 g cream* or rice milk or almond milk

Remove stems and core, cut in pieces, cook until soft and strain through a sieve.
Mix in.
Beat stiff and garnish with the piping bag.
K = 182 E = 1 g F = 6 g CH = 29 g (= 2½ BU)

200. Apple compote
150 g apples
50 g water
10 g laevoral or sorbitol
cinnamon or
grated lemon peel

Peel, remove the core and cut into wedges.
Boil.
Add and cook the apples in this juice until soft.
Add.
K = 121 E = 0 g F = 0 g CH = 28 g (= 2½ BU)

---

[1] Agar-agar is plant-based jelly powder used for vegetable and fruit spreads, sauces and puddings etc. instead of animal gelatine.

201. Halved apples
100 g apples
100 g water
10 g laevoral or sorbitol
¼ cinnamon stalk
10 g quince, raspberry or currant jelly
(sweetened with laevoral or sorbitol)

Peel, halve, hollow.
Boil.
Add the apples to the juice in batches and cook slowly until soft, then remove with a skimmer and arrange on a flat plate with the cut surface facing upwards.
Use to fill the hollowed-out half apples.
K = 138 E = 0 g F = 0 g CH = 32 g (= 2½ BU)

202. Blueberry mash
200 g blueberries
15 g laevoral or sorbitol
diluted with a little water
8 g soy flour with a little water
5 g wholemeal bread cubes in
5 g butter

Wash and sort, then
cook for 5 to 10 min.
Mix, add to the berries, boil and serve.
Cook and pour over the berries.
K = 224 E = 5 g F = 6 g CH = 36 g (= 3 BU)

203. Rhubarb compote
200 g rhubarb
25 g laevoral or sorbitol
25 g water and
5 g soy flour

Wash and dice.
Add rhubarb and cook briefly until soft.
Mix, add and cook.
Remove the soft rhubarb with a skimmer and arrange.
Let the juice boil down a little or compact with a little soy flour, and pour over the rhubarb.
K = 166 E = 3 g F = 2 g CH = 35 g (= 3 BU)

204. Strawberry coupe
150 g strawberries
10 g laevoral or sorbitol
50 g cream* or almond puree

Mix the berries or strain them through a fine-meshed sieve.
Add to the mixture to sweeten.
Whip and mix carefully with fruit.
Garnish with whole berries.

NB: Other fruits can also be used in this way.
K = 228 E = 3 g F = 12 g CH = 25 g
(= 2 BU)

205. Junket with fruits
("Hansen" brand recipe)
200 g milk
8 g laevoral or sorbitol, mixed with grated lemon zest
½ junket tablet
5 g water
10 g fresh berries

Heat the milk and sweet juice to approx. 37 °C.
Crush and dissolve in water, then immediately pour into heated milk, stir quickly and pour into glasses.
If the junket is solid, let cool.
Arrange over the junket just before serving.
K = 167 E = 6 g F = 7 g CH = 18 g (= 1½ BU)

206. Stuffed apples
100 g apples
15 g hazelnuts, ground
15 g cream
10 g laevoral or sorbitol
1 grated lemon peel
3 g butter
7 g laevoral or sorbitol
25 g grape juice

Cut out the core and score the peels.
Mix everything, fill into the apples and place in dish.
Spread over the apples, fill in 1 cm high and bake in oven for 20–30 min.
K = 288 E = 3 g F = 15 g CH = 35 g (= 3 BU)

207. Apple hedgehog*
100 g apples
8 g almonds

Like half apple, recipe no. 201.
Peel, cut into fine pins and roast lightly in the oven.
Arrange the half apples on a flat plate with the cut surface facing downwards, like mounds, and spiked with almond pins.
Mix 25 g cream with a little grated lemon peel, beat until half stiff and pour around the apples.
K = 158 E = 2 g F = 10 g CH = 14 g (= 1 BU)

208. Orange crème
1 piece orange peel with
50 g water and
5 g agar-agar, powdered
100 g orange juice
10 g lemon juice
25 g laevoral or sorbitol
1 egg
50 g cream* or almond paste

Whisk well, heat slowly over low heat until the agar-agar is fully dissolved.
Mix with dissolved agar-agar.
Stir until fluffy and mix in the fruit cream.
Beat until stiff and carefully fold in, arrange and leave to stand an hour.
K = 300 E = 6 g F = 15 g CH = 35 g (= 3 BU)

209. Lemon cream (cold stirred)
1 piece lemon peel
50 g water and
5 g agar-agar, powdered
50 g lemon juice
20 g laevoral or sorbitol
1 egg
50 g cream* or almond paste

Like orange cream, recipe no. 208.
K = 250 E = 5 g F = 14 g CH = 24 g (= 2 BU)

210. "Chaudeau"
1 egg
10 g laevoral or sorbitol
50 g orange juice
10 g lemon juice

Mix everything well, place in lukewarm water bath, heat slowly and stir until fluffy.

NB: Add some orange juice if the cream gets too thick.
K = 102 E = 4 g F = 3 g CH = 16 g (= 1½ BU)

211. Almond milk sauce
100 g milk
15 g almonds, peeled, grated
10 g laevoral or sorbitol
5 g soy flour with
50 g water

Boil together.
Mix and stir into the boiling milk.
Mix the sauce well.

NB: Almond puree can also be used instead of almonds.
K = 220 E = 7 g F = 12 g CH = 18 g (= 1½ BU)

Teas

The recipes can be prepared by your pharmacist.

212. Bean shell tea
Mix 20 g bean shells with 3 dl cold water overnight, boil for 5 min in the morning, let steep a few minutes, strain.
Drink 1–2 cups per day. The taste can be improved by adding equal parts of vegetable bouillon.

213. Honeysuckle tea (according to Stirnadel)
The pharmacist will provide you with a tea mixture according to the following recipe:
Rp: Herba Galegae conc.
    Semen Galegae aa p. aqu.

Use one heaping teaspoon of the tea mixture per glass of water, set to cold, boil briefly, let steep for 10 min. Three cups a day before meals.

214. Indian kidney tea
Instructions are on the package.

215. Jambul tea blend
Fruct. Syzygii jambulanae 20.0
Rad.   Tormentilla
Hb.   Potentilla
Hb.   Serpylli
Rad.   Artemisiae aa 10.0
Fruct. Phaseoli sine sem.
Fol.   Myrtilli aa 20.0

Leave 1½ teaspoon in 2 glasses of water overnight, boil briefly and strain. 1 cup before the meal.

216. Diabetes tea (Diab. tea no. 8 Faken)
Rp: Herba Urticae conc.
      Herba Galega conc.
      Fol. Myrtilli conc.
      Legumin Phaseol conc.
      Rad. Taraxaci c. herba conc. aa.

Briefly boil 1 tablespoon per cup of water and let steep for 10 min. One cup before each meal.
These recipes can be used alternatingly so that the body does not become accustomed to the same stimulus.

Annex and tables for the diabetes diet

Fresh juice day

(only with medical prescription and supervision)

Fresh juice fasting (during bed rest) is the ideal radical measure to start the slimming treatment. A bed-juice day provides:
1. Strongest food restriction with relatively high intake of high-quality active ingredients 300–500 calories.
2. Best rest for the heart, locomotor, respiratory and digestive systems, i.e. energy saving in favour of the body's adjustment work.
3. Drainage, without which the subsequent breakdown of fat tissue cannot take place.
4. Valuable mental relaxation, distancing oneself from day-to-day problems and processing them.

The juice day should take place 1–2 days per week beat the beginning of a slimming cure.

The juice should be enjoyed freshly squeezed. Fruit and vegetables should be ripe and as fresh as possible, if possible biologically fertilised, i.e. with compost instead of chemical or fresh animal-based fertilisers. Fruit: all juicy, ripe fruit appropriate to the season; vegetables should always be a mixture of root, tuber and green leaves. If possible, wild herbs, stinging nettles, dandelions and the like should be added (see juice recipes on page 90). Depending on weight, or on the severity of the treatment, the fresh juice days can be carried out in different forms (preparation, nutrition table for fruit and vegetables, page 89).

Strict daily schedule

1. 8 am: 200 g fruit juice;
   noon: 200 g vegetable juice;
   6 pm: 200 g fruit juice; total 600 g.

   Strict bed juice day 517 calories, protein 6 g, fat 4 g, carbohydrates 110 g (= 9 BU).
2. Milder form of the fresh juice day:
   8 am: 200 g fruit juice;
   noon: 200 g vegetable juice;
   4 pm: 200 g fruit juice;
   8 pm: 200 g vegetable juice total 800 g.

   Milder bed juice day 540 calories, protein 9 g, fat 2 g, carbohydrates 118 g (= 10 BU).

In case of low overweight, the third, mildest form of juice day,
3. **full juice day** can be observed once a week:
   8 am: 200 g fruit juice and 150 g almond milk or skimmed yoghurt;
   noon: 150 g fruit juice and 150 g vegetable juice mixture and 150 g almond milk or skimmed yoghurt;
   6 pm: same as 8 am.

   Full juice day 581 calories, protein 18 g, fat 2 g, carbohydrates 112 g (= 10 BU).

MENUS BY SEASON

Note on menu design

Some lunch menus are quite rich. If the number of calories is to be kept low, e.g. 1600 calories per day, either omit the soups and desserts or halve the individual portions so that the number of calories is not substantially exceeded.

Examples of menu compilations below:

Winter menus

Breakfast
Müesli (apples and oranges)
Wholemeal bread or crispbread
Butter or quark
Tree nuts, almonds, hazelnuts, pine seeds
Herbal teas (rosehips, lime blossoms, peppermint)
sweetened with sorbitol or laevoral
or
Milk or yoghurt
For a change, serve porridge (with milk) instead of bread.

Dinner
As breakfast
Poss. with addition of
- raw vegetable dishes
- or cheese with potatoes in jacket
- or salad with a soft egg or scrambled eggs
- or lettuce with porridge
- or salad with Riz Créol etc.
- or soup

Lunch for one week
1st day:
- Fruits (citrus fruits, apples)
- Raw vegetables: Carrots and endive
Cooked meals:
- Oat groats soup
- Stachys, steamed
- Caraway potatoes

2nd day:
- Raw vegetables: Celery (celeriac) and red cabbage
Cooked meals:
- Chicory and corn slices
- Orange jelly

3rd day:
- Raw vegetables: Black salsify and tomatoes and endive
Cooked meals:
- Semolina soup
- Brussels sprouts,
- Mashed potatoes

4th day:
- Fruits
- Raw vegetables: Red beets and sauerkraut
Cooked meals:
- Fennel and Riz-Créol
- Apple mash

5th day:
- Fruits
- Raw vegetables: Cauliflower and spinach
Cooked meals:
- Bouillon with strips of pancake
- Celery vegetables and potato sticks

6th day:
- Fruits
- Raw vegetables: Jerusalem artichoke and lettuce
Cooked meals:
- Vegetable soup
- Leek vegetables and potato cakes

7th day:
- Fruits
- Raw vegetables: Fennel and lamb's lettuce
Cooked meals:
- Lettuce
- Soy pasta and tomato sauce
- Stuffed apples

Spring menus

Breakfast and dinner as pp. 124

Lunch for one week
1ˢᵗ day:
- Fruits (strawberries, apples, citrus fruits)
- Raw vegetables: Radishes and cress and lettuce

Cooked meals:
- Spring soup
- Spinach
- Sesame potatoes

2ⁿᵈ day:
- Fruits
- Raw vegetables: Parsnip and tomatoes and lamb's lettuce

Cooked meals:
- Courgettes and risotto
- Rhubarb compote

3ʳᵈ day:
- Fruits
- Raw vegetables: Red beets and cucumbers and lettuce

Cooked meals:
- Spinach soup
- Cauliflower and parsley potatoes

4ᵗʰ day:
- Fruits
- Raw vegetables: Tomatoes and chicory

Cooked meals:
- Chervil soup
- Spinach – whole leaves
- Soy pasta

5ᵗʰ day:
- Fruits
- Raw vegetables: Celery (celeriac) and dandelion

Cooked meals:
- Kohlrabi and potato slices with spinach and egg
- Cream of curd cheese

6ᵗʰ day:
- Fruits
- Raw vegetables: Carrot and cress and lettuce

Cooked meals:
- Tomato vegetables
- Oat flake roasts

7ᵗʰ day:
- Fruits
- Raw vegetables: Cauliflower and lettuce

Cooked meals:
- Vegetable plate (tomatoes, celery (celeriac), carrots)
- Potato puree
- Strawberries with whipped cream

Summer menus

Breakfast and dinner as pp. 124

Lunch for one week
1ˢᵗ day:
- Fruits (apples, currants, raspberries, peaches, apricots)
- Raw vegetables: Horseradish, tomatoes, head lettuce

Cooked meals:
- Stuffed paprika with rice
- Beans

2ⁿᵈ day:
- Fruits
- Raw vegetables: Celery (celeriac), spinach, head lettuce

Cooked meals:
- Cabbage stems with cheese and potatoes in peel
- Stuffed melons (with fruit salad)

3ʳᵈ day:
- Fruits
- Raw vegetables: Salad niçoise (mixed salad)

Cooked meals:
- Spinach and quark potatoes

4ᵗʰ day:
- Fruits
- Raw vegetables: Red beets and courgettes and cress

Cooked meals:
- Potato soup
- Hirsotto with vegetables

5th day:
- Fruits
- Raw vegetables: Cauliflower and cucumber and lettuce

Cooked meals:
- Artichokes and remoulade sauce
- Mashed potatoes (puree)

6th day:
- Fruits
- Raw vegetables: Carrot and fennel and lettuce

Cooked meals:
- Chopped spinach
- Omelettes
- Apricot junket

7th day:
- Fruits
- Raw vegetables: Kohlrabi and tomatoes

Cooked meals:
- Bean soup
- Courgettes and risotto with bell peppers

Autumn menus

Breakfast and dinner as pp. 124

Lunch for one week

1st day:
- Fruits (apples, pears, plums, peaches, citrus fruits, blackberries), raw vegetables: beetroot, courgette and endive

Cooked meals:
- Bouillon with egg
- Beans and stewed potatoes

2nd day:
- Fruits
- Raw vegetables: bread rolls topped with raw vegetables and lettuce

Cooked meals:
- Baked cauliflower and aubergine with tomato sauce

3rd day:
- Fruits
- Raw vegetables: Celery (celeriac) and sauerkraut

Cooked meals:
- Endives and potato plums
- Orange brawn heads

4th day:
- Fruits
- Raw vegetables: Tomatoes stuffed with celery salad and head lettuce

Cooked meals:
- Cabbage soup with potatoes
- Fennel and cheese slices

5th day:
- Fruits
- Raw vegetables: Cauliflower and lamb's lettuce and head lettuce

Cooked meals:
- Clear vegetable soup
- Red beets and cream potatoes

6th day:
- Fruits
- Raw vegetables: Russian salad garnished with cucumber, tomatoes and cress

Cooked meals:
- Leaf spinach and soy omelettes

7th day:
- Fruits
- Raw vegetables: Radish and spinach and endive

Cooked meals:
- Lettuce garnished with peas
- Potato pancakes
- Stuffed peaches or apples

Calculated daily menus for the diabetes diet (1200–2100 K)

Legend:

Gram	g	
Calories	C	(fuel energy)
Protein	P	in grams
Fat	F	in grams
Carbohydrates	CH	in grams
Bread units	BU	12 g CH = 1 Bread unit

Table III Bircher Whole Foods 1200 calories* diet

Breakfast and dinner					
	C	P g	F g	CH g	BU
Müesli					
3 g oat flakes	13.5	0.45	0.15	2.4	
3 tablespoons water	–	–	–	–	
7 g lemon juice	2.0	–	–	0.5	
38 g yoghurt	28.0	1.8	1.4	1.7	
7 g fruit concentrate	18.0	–	–	4.5	
150 g apples	78.5	0.45	0.45	18.2	
15 g nuts	70.0	3.0	5.4	1.8	
= 220 g	210.0	5.7	7.4	29.1	2.4
plus add to müesli					
20 g wholemeal bread	51.0	1.5	–	10.0	
5 g butter	38.0	–	4.0	–	
125 g fruits	53.0	0.9	0.2	13.6	
25 g quark	22.0	4.2	0.2	0.5	
	164.0	6.6	4.4	24.1	2
for breakfast and dinner each	374.0	12.3	11.9	53.3	approx. 4 ½

* Values based on 100 g edible share

Lunch					
	C	P g	F g	CH g	BU
100 g fruits	50.0	0.7	0.2	10.8	
Sauce for raw vegetables					
30 g yoghurt	22.2	1.4	1.1	1.3	
10 g lemon juice some onion juice, 1 knife tip of dried herbs, mixed well	3.0	–	–	0.7	
Raw food					
100 g head lettuce	15.0	1.4	0.2	2.0	
100 g cauliflower	26.0	2.0	0.1	4.0	
50 g cucumber	3.0	0.3	–	0.3	
½ egg	36.0	3.0	2.5	0.2	
	155.2	8.8	4.1	19.3	
Cooked vegetables (interchangeable)					
200 g tomatoes	37.6	2.0	0.4	6.6	
50 g onions 1 tablespoon parsley, baked on a greased baking tray	22.6	0.6	0.1	4.8	
5 g oil	46.0	–	5.0	–	
	106.2	2.6	5.5	11.4	
100 g potatoes in jacket	85.0	2.0	0.1	18.9	
50 g low-fat curd cheese	44.1	8.5	0.3	1.0	
	129.1	10.5	0.4	19.9	
Lunch: total	390.0	21.9	10.0	50.7	approx. 4
Snack between meals: 150 g yoghurt	109.0	7.2	5.6	6.7	
Total intake per day	**1247.0**	**53.8**	**39.4**	**164.0**	**approx. 13**

Table IV Bircher Whole Foods 1600 calories* diet

Breakfast and dinner					
	C	P g	F g	CH g	BU
Müesli					
5 g oat flakes	18.1	0.6	0.25	3.2	
50 g water	–	–	–	–	
10 g lemon juice	3.0	–	–	0.7	
50 g yoghurt	37.0	2.4	1.9	2.2	
20 g laevulose	48.0	–	–	12.0	
200 g apples	104.8	0.6	0.6	24.2	
20 g nuts	93.0	4.0	7.2	2.4	
Total	303.9	7.6	9.9	44.7	
With					
20 g wholemeal bread	51.0	1.5	–	10.0	
15 g butter	76.0	–	8.0	–	
125 g fruits	53.0	0.9	0.2	13.6	
50 g quark	44.0	8.5	0.3	1.0	
Total	224.0	10.9	8.5	24.6	
Breakfast and dinner, each	527.9	18.5	18.4	69.3	approx. 6
One snack between meals					
150 g yoghurt	109.0	7.2	5.6	6.7	approx. ½
Lunch					
100 g fruits	49.0	0.7	0.2	10.8	
30 g yoghurt	21.2	1.4	1.1	1.3	
10 g lemon	3.0	–	–	0.7	
some onion juice, 1 knife tip of dried herbs					
50 g head lettuce	7.5	0.7	0.1	1.0	
50 g cucumber	3.0	0.3	–	0.3	
100 g cauliflower	26.0	2.0	0.1	4.0	
½ egg mixed in sauce	36.0	3.0	2.5	0.2	
Total	145.7	8.1	4.0	18.3	

* Values based on 100 g edible share

Lunch					
	C	P g	F g	CH g	BU
Boiled vegetables (can BU replaced by other vegetables)					
200 g tomatoes	39.0	2.0	0.4	6.6	
50 g onions	22.6	0.6	0.1	4.8	
1 tablespoon parsley					
Bake on a greased baking tray:					
10 g oil	92.0	–	10.0	–	
Total	153.6	2.6	10.5	11.4	
100 g potatoes in the peel	85.0	2.0	0.1	18.9	
50 g low-fat curd cheese	44.1	8.5	0.3	1.0	
Total	129.1	10.5	0.4	19.9	
Subtotal for lunch	428.4	21.2	14.9	49.6	approx. 4
Total intake per day	1593.0	65.4	57.3	194.9	approx. 16

Table V Bircher Whole Foods 2100 calories* diet

Breakfast and dinner					
	C	P g	F g	CH g	BU
Müesli:					
5 g oat flakes	18.1	0.6	0.25	3.2	
30 g cream	73.5	1.1	6.9	1.1	
10 g lemon juice	3.0	–	–	0.7	
50 g yoghurt	37.0	2.4	1.9	2.2	
20 g laevulose	48.0	–	–	12.0	
20 g nuts	104.8	0.6	0.6	24.2	
200 g apples	93.0	4.0	7.2	2.4	
Total	377.4	8.7	16.8	45.8	
With					
20 g wholemeal bread	47.0	1.5	–	10.0	
15 g butter	114.0	–	12.6	–	
75 quark	66.0	12.7	0.4	1.5	
10 g laevulose	24.0	–	–	6.0	
180 g fruits (Part of the fruit may be eaten for snacks.)	90.0	1.3	0.4	19.4	
Total	341.0	15.5	13.1	36.9	

Breakfast and dinner					
	C	P g	F g	CH g	BU
Breakfast and dinner, each	718.4	24.2	29.3	82.7	approx. 7
Two snacks between meals					
150 g yoghurt	109.0	7.2	5.6	6.7	
150 g milk	109.0	7.2	5.6	6.7	
Total	218.0	14.4	11.2	13.4	
Lunch, as in the diet for 1600 calories					
	428.0	21.2	14.8	49.6	approx. 4
Total intake per day	2082.0	84.0	85.2	228.4	approx. 19

Table VI Raw food diet with 1200 calories

Breakfast					
	C	P g	F g	CH g	BU
Müesli:					
10 g laevulose	41.0	–	–	10.0	
20 g cream	60.0	0.4	6.1	0.5	
100 g apples	54.0	0.3	0.3	12.1	
25 g yoghurt	18.0	1.2	1.0	1.1	
10 g lemon	3.0	–	–	0.7	
100 g fruits	54.0	0.3	0.3	12.1	
20 nuts	93.0	4.0	7.2	2.4	
	323.0	6.2	14.9	38.9	approx. 3
Lunch					
100 g fruits	54.0	0.3	0.3	12.1	
20 g almonds	120.0	3.6	10.0	3.0	
100 g cauliflower	26.0	2.0	0.2	4.0	
50 g cucumber	3.0	0.3	–	0.3	
50 g salad	7.0	0.7	0.1	1.0	
10 g cream	30.0	0.2	3.0	0.3	
10 g oil	92.0	–	9.9	0.05	
15 g lemon juice	4.0	–	–	1.0	
10 g quark	9.0	1.7	0.1	0.2	
	345.0	8.8	23.6	21.9	approx. 2

Dinner					
	C	P g	F g	CH g	BU
As breakfast	323.0	6.2	14.9	38.9	
With					
50 g salad	7.0	0.7	0.1	1.0	
50 g chicory	18.0	0.6	0.1	1.1	
Cream, oil, lemon juice and quark	135.0	1.9	13.0	1.5	
	473.0	9.4	28.1	42.5	approx. 3
Total value	1141.0	24.4	66.6	103.3	approx. 8

Table VII Raw food diet with 1900 calories

Breakfast					
	C	P g	F g	CH g	BU
Müesli					
10 g laevulose	41.0	–	–	10.0	
40 g cream	121.0	0.9	12.2	1.0	
200 g apples	107.0	0.6	0.6	24.2	
50 g yoghurt	37.0	2.4	1.9	2.2	
10 g lemon	3.0	–	–	0.7	
250 g fruits	123.0	1.8	0.5	27.1	
20 g nuts	93.0	4.0	7.2	2.4	
	525.0	9.7	22.4	67.7	approx. 6
150 g yoghurt	109.0	7.2	5.7	6.6	approx. ½
Lunch					
250 g fruits	123.0	1.8	0.5	27.1	
20 g almonds	120.0	3.6	10.0	3.0	
100 g cauliflower	26.0	2.0	0.2	4.0	
50 g cucumbers	3.0	0.3	–	0.3	
50 g salad	7.0	0.7	0.1	1.0	
10 g cream quark	9.0	1.7	0.1	0.2	
10 g cream	30.0	0.2	3.0	0.3	
20 g oil	185.0	–	19.9	0.1	
15 g lemon juice	4.0	–	–	1.1	
	507.0	10.3	33.8	37.1	approx. 3

Dinner					
	C	P g	F g	CH g	BU
As breakfast	525.0	9.7	22.4	67.7	
With					
50 g salad	7.0	0.7	0.1	1.0	
50 g chicory	8.0	0.6	0.1	1.1	
10 g cream	30.0	0.2	3.0	0.3	
20 g oil	185.0	–	19.9	0.1	
15 g lemon juice	4.0	–	–	1.1	
	759.0	11.2	45.5	71.3	approx. 6
Total value	1900.0	38.4	107.4	182.7	approx. 15

Table VIII Composition of the most common foods

Calories and protein content, values expressed per 100 g edible share

Vegetables (non-fat) calories and protein content

2.5 g carbohydrates in 100 g	C1	P*
Chicory	12	1
Kale	12	1
Cucumber	12	1
Spinach juice	12	1
Watercress	11	1
Endives	12	2
Lamb's lettuce	20	2
Head lettuce	12	2
Chard	25	2
Asparagus	15	2
White mushrooms	25	3
5.0 g carbohydrates in 100 g	**C***	**P***
Aubergines	25	1
Celery	25	1
Garden cress	50	1
Carrot juice	25	1
Pumpkin	25	1
Leek	25	1

5.0 g carbohydrates in 100 g	C*	P*
Radishes	25	1
Rhubarb	25	1
Red cabbage	25	1
Sauerkraut	25	1
Tomatoes	25	1
Tomato juice	25	1
Canned tomatoes	25	1
White cabbage	25	1
Cauliflower	25	1
10 g carbohydrates in 100 g	**C***	**P* g**
Green beans	25	1
Stalk celery	50	2
Broccoli	25	3
Spinach	25	3
Porcini mushrooms	25	3
Carrots	25	1
Pumpkin	25	1
Red beet	50	1
Celery	50	1
Artichokes	50	2

1 Values based on 100 g edible share

10 g carbohydrates in 100 g	C1*	P* g
Brussels sprouts	50	4
Truffles	50	5
Green peas	50	3
canned		1
15 g carbohydrates in 100 g	**C***	**P***
Parsnip	69	1
Black salsify	66	1
Jerusalem artichoke	74	2
Horseradish	76	2.8
Green peas	93	7
20 g carbohydrates in 100 g	**C***	**P***
Potato	85	2
Fresh sweet corn	107	3

Above 20 g carbohydrates in 100 g (calories, protein, fat and carbohydrate content)	C	P g	F g	CH2* g
Sweet potatoes	124	1		26.6
White beans	352	21	2	57.6
Ripe peas	370	23	1	60.7
Lentils	303	22	1	49
Soy beans	445	37	18	26.8
Soy flakes	469	37	21	26.4
Dried porcini mushrooms	74	20	3	43.6

Fruits (not containing fat), calories and protein content

5 g carbohydrates in 100 g	C1	P* g
Papaya	9	0.2
Watermelon	28	0.6
Lemon	28	0.7
Lemon juice	24	0.3

10 g carbohydrates in 100 g	C*	P* g
Acerola	39	0.2
Apples	50	0.3
Apple juice	47	0.1
Apricot	54	0.9
Pear	59	0.5
Blackberries	48	42
Strawberries	39	0.9
Grapefruits	32	0.7
Grapefruit juice	28	0.6
Raspberries	40	1.2
Elderberries	46	2.5
Currants, red	37	1.0
Currants, black	46	1.0
Currants, white	38	0.9
Tangerines	43	0.9
Oranges	54	0.9
Orange juice	47	0.8
Peaches	46	0.7
Plums	53	0.7
Cranberries	46	0.3
Gooseberries	44	0.8
15 g carbohydrates in 100 g	**C***	**P* g**
Pineapples	57	0.5
Figs	73	1.3
Cherries, sour	60	0.2
Cherries, sweet	64	0.8
Blueberries	62	0.6
Mirabelles	67	0.7
Greengage	72	0.8
Grapes	74	0.7
Plums	36	0.7
20 g carbohydrates in 100 g	**C***	**P* g**
Bananas	90	1.1
Rosehip jelly	102	3.6
Grape juice	74	1.0

---

1 Values based on 100 g edible share

Dried fruits

	C	P g	F g	CH1 g
Apples	279	1.4	1.6	65
Apricots	300	5.0	0.4	66
Dates	305	18.0	0.5	73
Figs	272	3.5	1.3	61
Chestnuts	211	3.0	2.0	43
Peaches	282	3.0	0.6	66
Plums	293	2.3	0.6	69
Raisins	305	2.3	0.5	71

Bread

	C	P g	F g	CH* g
Graham bread	250	8.4	1.0	48
Crispbread	383	10.1	1.4	77
Pumpernickel	247	6.8	0.9	49
Wholemeal rye bread	239	7.3	1.2	46
Stonemason's bread	254	7.6	1.0	50
Wholemeal wheat bread	241	7.5	0.9	47

Nuts

	C	P g	F g	CH*g
Roasted peanuts	631	26.5	47	19
Hazelnuts	690	14	62	13
Coconut	399	41	36	10
Almonds	651	18	54	16
Poppy seed	467	14	37	16
Brazil nuts	714	14	67	7
Pine seeds	610	20	50	20
Walnuts	705	15	63	13
Swiss stone pine seed	562	4	49	22

* Values based on 100 g edible share

Milk, dairy products and fats

	C	P g	F g	CH* g
Butter	755	0.7	81	–
Buttermilk	36	3.5	0.5	4
Buttermilk powder	384	33	2	55
Camembert cheese	301	18	23	1.8
Double cream fresh cheese	354	14.6	–	1.9
Edam cheese	238	26.1	23.6	3.5
Emmental cheese	417	30	3.4	27
Gervais cheese	414	13	38	1.7
Yoghurt	74	4.8	3.7	4.5
Sweetened condensed milk	335	8	8.8	55
Condensed milk unsweetened	141	7	7.7	9.8
Condensed skimmed milk	277	10	0.2	58
Cow's milk	68	3.4	–	5
Low-fat cheese, average	222	36	6.5	3.5
Skimmed milk	35	3	0.1	4.8
Skimmed milk powder	368	35	1	52
Lean quark	88	17	0.6	1.8
Whey, sweet	24	0.8	0.2	4.6
Whey powder	346	12	1	71
Parmesan cheese	410	36	26	3.5
Quark	97	17	1.2	4
Cream cheese	417	16	37	1.7
Roquefort cheese	419	24	33	3.7
Cream	302	2.2	30	3
Processed cheese	305	14	23.6	6.1
Whole milk powder	503	25	26	38
Peanut paste	641	26.1	48	19

	C	P g	F g	CH* g
Coconut oil	925	18	99	–
Corn oil	930	–	100	–
Margarine	733	0.51	78.4	–
Olive oil	927	–	99.6	–
Palmin	902	–	97.0	–

Cereals (grains)

	C	P g	F g	CH*g
Cornflakes	382	7.7	0.6	82
Barley	370	10.6	2.1	72
Barley, peeled	330	8.0	1.6	69
Barley groats	368	8.5	1.5	75
Barley flour	369	10.6	1.9	72
Wholemeal oats	387	12.6	7.1	63
Oats, peeled	351	11.0	6.0	61
Oat flakes	402	13.8	6.6	66
Porridge	399	13.9	5.8	67
Oatmeal	410	14.9	7.5	66
Millet, peeled	382	10.6	3.9	70.7

	C	P g	F g	CH*g
Corn, whole grain	375	9.2	3.8	71
Maize meal	376	8.9	2.8	74
Polished rice	368	7.0	0.6	75
Unpolished rice	371	7.4	2.2	75
Rice flour	311	7.2	0.65	79
Rye, wholemeal	359	11.6	1.7	69
Rye sprouts	404	42.0	11.2	26
Rye flour	363	8.6	1.2	–
Sunflower seed flour	359	37.0	10.6	36
Wheat, whole grain	363	11.7	2.0	69
Wheat semolina	326	7.0	0.2	72
Wheat sprouts	400	26.6	9.2	46
Wheat bran	361	16.0	4.6	51
Wheat flour	368	10.6	1.0	74
Pioneer rice sprouts	–	20.3	24.7	–

---

* Values based on 100 g edible share

Table of glycaemic index and glycaemic charge

The glycaemic index shows how quickly and how high the blood sugar will climb when a certain food is eaten. It is expressed in % of the rise caused by the same amount of glucose.

The glycaemic charge is calculated by taking the glycaemic index and multiplying it by the content of pure carbohydrates. If a food has a high glycaemic index and consists mainly of pure carbohydrates, it has a very high glycaemic charge. If it mostly contains pure carbohydrates that are converted into glucose, the food will need a lot of insulin to enter the cells and allow the blood sugar level settle again.

Only those carbohydrates that are converted into glucose (and therefore need insulin to BU absorbed into the cells) will produce a blood glucose increase after a meal. Other sugar types, such as those in fruits and vegetables, that are not converted to glucose (fructose, sorbitol etc.) do not increase the glycaemic index and do not require insulin. The glycaemic index therefore provides the best information for calculating the insulin required to ingest a particular food.

The glycaemic charge load contains all pure carbohydrates, including those that do not need insulin to BU processed, due to multiplication of the glycaemic index with the content of all pure carbohydrates. Therefore it is less suitable for calculating insulin requirements than the glycaemic index. On the other hand, it has proved useful to take this into account, as it has been shown that foods with a high glycaemic charge have an unfavourable effect on the fat metabolism disorder by increasing the triglyceride level.

Concerning diabetes, foods that have a low glycaemic index and a low glycaemic charge are best, while being good food integrals. Their carbohydrate content should be mostly of fructose and other sugar types that do not need insulin, and the glucose content should be that which can only be broken down slowly during digestion. These are the uncooked fruits, vegetables, whole grains and nuts of raw food.

Foods	Glycaemic index in%	Glycaemic charge
Amaranth	30	< 10
Pineapples	59	6
Bottled pineapple juice	46	6
Apples	38	5
Apple, dried	29	16
Bottled apple juice, clear	40	5
Apple juice, naturally clouded	37	4
Apricots, fresh	57	4
Apricots, dried	31	14
Artichokes	20	2
Aubergines	10	< 10
Avocado	20	< 10
Baguette, white bread	70	36
Bananas	52	10
Pears	38	9
Sponge cake	46	26
Green salads	10	0
Pretzel	83	48
Broccoli	10	< 10
Beans, black	42	8
Beans, cooked white	48	5
Green beans (mung beans)	38	?
Beans (kidney)	28	5
Buckwheat	54	11
Bulgur, cooked	48	8
Buttermilk, natural	< 10	< 10
Shortbread biscuit	51	37
Cornflakes	81	70
Couscous	65	15
Dried dates	103	69
Ice cream, full cream	61	13
Peas (fresh)	40	4

Foods	Glycaemic index in%	Glycaemic charge
Strawberries	40	1
Figs, fresh	40	?
Figs, dried	61	21
Fruit bread	47	24
Bottled vegetable juice	43	2
Grapefruit	25	2
Bottled grapefruit juice	48	4
Barley	43	12
Gluten-free light bread	76	38
Semolina	65	4
Green spelt	55	?
Oat flakes	59	36
Oat bran bread	47	28
Oatmeal bread	65	41
Oat porridge	60	8
Oat bran	55	28
Hamburger bread	85	31
Millet, cooked	71	17
Honey	55	40
Yoghurt, natural	36	2
Fruit yoghurt, sugared	40	6
Fruit yoghurt, sweetener	14	1
Yoghurt drink	38	6
Persimmon	50	8
Jam (marmalade)	51	34
Carrots, raw	47	4
Carrots, cooked	85	3
Bottled carrot juice	43	4
Baked potatoes	85	17
Potatoes, boiled	78	11
Potatoes, gnocchi	68	18
Potato mash	74	10

Foods	Glycaemic index in%	Glycaemic charge
Potato mash from powder	85	11
Potatoes, new	57	8
Potatoes, French fries	75	15
Potatoes, crisps	54	23
Potatoes, sweet potatoes	61	11
Chick peas, cooked	38	6
Cherries	22	2
Kiwi	50	5
Bran bread	50	10
Crispbread, fibre-rich	59	35
Rye crispbread	64	41
Garlic	10	< 10
cabbage	10	0
Kohlrabi, cooked	70	5
Rutabaga, yellow	70	7
Crackers	67	38
Pumpkin, cooked	75	4
Leek	10	< 10
Lentils, green cooked	30	3
Lentils, red cooked	26	3
Lean quark	10	1
Corn (sweet corn)	54	11
Maizemeal (polenta)	69	6
Corn, popcorn	72	40
Mango	51	7
Mars bar	65	43
Melon (honeydew melon)	65	3
Horseradish	35	< 10
Milk, partially skimmed	32	2
Milk, whole	27	1
Whey, natural	< 10	< 10
Milk bread roll (Weggli)	63	34
Müesli flakes, industrial	49	33
Muffin	53	30
Nutella	33	20
Natural yoghurt	35	1–5
Nuts (average)	25	1–5
Nuts, cashew	22	3
Nuts, peanuts	15	2
Nectarine	30	< 10
Fruit (average value)	35–45	3–10
Oranges	42	4
Bottled orange juice	50	5
Papaya	59	8
Parsnip	85	3
Boiled potatoes (boiled)	65	10
Paprika	10	< 10
Peach	42	4
Plums	39	4
Plums, dried	29	16
Mushrooms	15	0
Pumpernickel	50	20
Quinoa	35	?
Radishes	30	< 10
Basmati rice	58	15
Jasmine scented rice	109	31
Long-grain rice	56	16
Rice Krispies (Kellogg's)	82	71
Parboiled rice	47	11
Risotto rice	69	24
White rice	64	15
Radish	35	1
Rice Krispies	82	71
Rye grains (whole)	35	26

Foods	Glycaemic index in%	Glycaemic charge
Wholemeal rye bread	50	30
Rye sourdough bread	53	21
Rye wholemeal bread	58	27
Raisins	64	47
Beetroot, cooked	65	3
Sauerkraut	15	0
Chocolate whole milk	43	24
Celery tubers, cooked	85	2
Soy bean, cooked	18	1
Soybean sprouts	20	< 10
Asparagus	15	0
Raisins	56	42
Pasta (average)	60	40

Foods	Glycaemic index in%	Glycaemic charge
Pasta soy glass noodles	33	8
Pasta egg noodles	40	10
Pasta rice noodles	61	13
Pasta spaghetti al dente	44	12
Pasta spaghetti soft	61	15
Pasta wholemeal al dente	37	9
Wheat semolina (white)	60	7
Wheat sprouts	60	9
Wheat coarse meal	75	50
White wheat bread	70	33
Lemons	15	< 10
Courgette	10	< 10
Onions	10	< 10

List of recipes

Almond milk	90	Buckwheat meal	115
Almond milk sauce	121	Butter, health-food store vegetable	
American tomatoes	101	fats and oils	91
Apple compote	119		
Apple hedgehog	120	Cabbage, chopped	105
Apple mash	119	Cabbage or white cabbage, sautéed	104
Apples, halved	119	Cabbage soup with potatoes	96
Apples, stuffed	120	Cabbage stems	98
Aritchokes, Jerusalem	100	Cabbage stems or "false asparagus"	98
Artichokes	103	Caraway or sesame seed potatoes	109
Artichokes, roman	103	Cardoon	99
Artichokes, sautéed	103	Carrot soup	94
Asparagus	103	Carrots, sautéed	99
Aubergine	102	Cauliflower	104
Aubergines	102	Cauliflower polonaise	104
Aubergines, stuffed	103	Cauliflower soup	94
		Celery salad with mayonnaise	108
Baked potatoes	109	Celery, sautéed	99
Basic spreads	108	Celery soup	95
Beans, dried	99	Celery stalk	98
Beans, green	99	Cereal Dishes	112
Bean shell tea	121	Chaudeau	121
Beans, white, with Tomatoes	106	Cheese casserole	117
Béchamel sauce	117	Cheese sandwiches	116
Beetroot vegetables	100	Chervil soup	95
Bell pepper sauce	118	Chicory	98
Bell peppers, green or yellow, sautéed	102	Chicory polonaise	98
Bell peppers, stuffed	102	Corn on the cob	104
Bircher müesli	84	Courgettes, 1st option	101
Bircher müesli with almond puree	84	Courgettes, 2nd option	101
Bircher müesli with cream	84	Cream dressing	87
Bircher müesli with various fruits	85	Cream potatoes	110
Bircher müesli with yoghurt	84		
Black salsify, sautéed	99	Desserts	118
Blueberry mash	120	Diabetes tea	122
Bouillon potatoes	110	Dressings for raw vegetables	
Bouillon, vegetable	92	and salads	87
Broccoli (a kind of cauliflower)	104	Dried beans	99
Broth, vegetable	92		
Brussels sprouts, sautéed	104	Egg custard	92
Buckwheat groats	115	Endive vegetables	98

141

Fennel	98	Onion vegetables	106
Fruit jelly	119	Orange crème	121
Fruit juices	90		
Fruit salad	119	Parsley potatoes	110
		Peperonata	102
Gold cubes	93	Pine nut milk	90
Green beans	99	Plant milk types	90
Gruel soup	94	Polenta	114
		Potato cakes	111
Herbal omelettes	116	Potato dishes	109
Herbal sauce	117	Potato dumplings	111
Hirsotto	115	Potatoes in jacket	109
Hirsotto with vegetables	115	Potatoes "Schloss"	112
Honeysuckle tea	121	Potatoes with kale (stew)	112
Horseradish sauce	118	Potatoes with tomatoes	110
Hot food	91	Potato pancakes	111
		Potato puree	110
Indian kidney tea	121	Potato salad, 1st option	107
		Potato salad, 2nd option	107
Jambul tea blend	121	Potato salad with cucumbers	107
Japanese rice	112	Potato slices with spinach	112
Junket with fruits	120	Potato soup	95
		Potato soup with leeks	95
Kale	105	Potato soup with soy flour	96
Kohlrabi, steamed	105	Potato wedges (cooked raw)	112
		Princess potatoes	111
Leek vegetables	106		
Lemon cream (cold stirred)	121	Quark potatoes	109
Lettuce	97		
Lyon potatoes	111	Raw vegetables and salads	85
		Red cabbage	105
Maize porridge	114	Rhubarb compote	120
Maize slices	115	Rice dishes	112
Mashed potato	110	Rice gratin with tomatoes	114
Mayonnaise dressing	87	Rice ring or rice head	114
Mayonnaise dressing with soy flour		Rice salad	107
instead of egg	87	Rice soup, clear	93
Mayonnaise made with soy		Rice soup, italian style	93
instead of egg	118	Rice with courgettes	113
Mayonnaise sauce	118	Rice with peas	113
Minestrone	96	Rice with spinach	114
Mixed vegetables	106	Risotto	112
Müesli with berries or stone fruit	85	Risotto with bel peppers	113
		Riz Creol	113
Oil dressing	87	Riz Créol with vegetables	113
Omelettes, French	116	Roasted oat flakes	115
Omelettes, French, with tomatoes	116	Roast potatoes	111
Onion sauce	117	Russian eggs	108
		Russian salad	107

Saffron rice	113	Strawberry coupe	120
Sago soup with vegetable add-ins	93	Stuffing for "stuffed vegetables"	106
Salad Niçoise	107		
Salads of cooked vegetables	106	Teas	121
Sandwiches	108	Tomatoes à la Provence	101
Sauerkraut	105	Tomatoes, baked	100
Sauerkraut salad	88	Tomatoes, stuffed	100
Semolina dumplings	93	Tomatoes with cheese slices	100
Sesame cream	91	Tomatoes with scrambled eggs	101
Sesame frappé	91	Tomato rice	113
Sesame milk	91	Tomato sauce, 1st option	117
Soup add-ins	92	Tomato sauce, 2nd option	117
Soups	92	Tomato soup, 1st option	94
Soup, spinach or chard	94	Tomato soup, 2nd option	94
Sour white cabbage	105	Tomato vegetables	100
Soy milk (Molat)	91		
Soy omelettes	116	Vegetable bouillon	92
Soy soup	93	Vegetable brawn	108
Spinach, chopped, 2nd option	97	Vegetable juices	90
Spinach or chard soup	94	Vegetables	96
Spinach pudding	116	Vinaigrette	118
Spinach, whole leaves, 1st option	97		
Spinach, whole leaves, 2nd option	97	White beans with tomatoes	106
Spinach, whole leaves, 3rd option	97	White mushroom sauce,	
Spring soup	95	for refinement	118
Sprouted cereal grains	89		
Stachys	104	Yoghurt dressing	87
Strawberries in lemon juice	119		

Literatur

1. IDF Pressemitteilung, "Diabetes epidemic out of control", Presseaussendung, 4 Dec 2006, https://web.Archive.Org/web/200911120194932/ http:/www.idf.org/node/1354.
2. Danaei, G. et al., "National, regional and global trends in fasting plasma glucose and diabetes precalence since 1980: systematic analysis of health examination surveys and epidemiological studies with 370 country-years and 2.7 million participants" Lancet, vol 378, no 9785, July 2011, pp 31–40, PMID 21705069.
3. IDF Diabetes Atlas, 4th edition, IDF 2013 diabetesatlas.org (http://www.diabetesatlas.org/).
4. Internationale Diabetesfederation: "Leitlinie für die Postprandiale Diabeteseinstellung", (http://www.idf.org/webdata/docs/German_GMPG %20Final%20110108.pdf) ss.2008, viewed on 30 July 2011.
5. WHO: "Definition and diagnosis of diabetes mellitus and intermediate hyperglycemia", D (http://www.who.int/diabetes/publications/ Definition%20and%20diagnosis%20of%20 diabetes_new.pdf), viewed on 19 Feb 2011.
6. Holterhus, P.M. et al., "Diagnostik, Therapie, Verlaufskontrolle des Diabetes mellitus im Kindes- und Jugendalter" (http://www.deutsche-diabetes-gesellschaft.de/redaktion/mitteilungen/leitlinien/ EBL_Kindesalter_2010.pdf),PDF,deutsche-diabetes-gesellschaft.de, 2010, p 18 (viewed on, 20 Feb 2011).
7. Kerne, W. et al., "Definition, Klassifikation und Diagnostik des Diabetes mellitus" (http://www. deutsche-diabetes-gesellschaft.de/fileadmin/ Redakteur/Leitlinien/Praxisleitlinien/2012/DuS_ S2-12_Praxisempfehlungen_Kerner-Brueckel_S84-87.pdf)(PDF;846 kB), DDG, 1 Oct 2012, viewed on 1 April 2013.
8. Boeck, G. et al., Prüfungswissen Physikum, Thieme-Verlag, Stuttgart 2009, ISBN 978-3-13-152131-6, p 521.
9. Concannon, P. et al., "Genetics of type 1 A diabetes", New Engl J Medicine, 360 (16), April 2009, pp 1646–54, PMID 19369670.
10. Nejntsev, S. et al., "Localization of type I diabetes susceptibility to the MHC class I genes HLA-B and HLA-A" Nature, vol 450 (7171), Dec 2007, pp 887–892, PMID 18004301.
11. Ziegler, A.G. et al., "Kaiserschnitt erhöht das Risiko für Typ-1-Diabetes: Ergebinisse aus der BABYDIAB-Studie" (http://cme.medlearning.de/ dzkf/kaiserschnitt_erhoetes_risiko_fuer_diabetes/ pdf/CME_Beitrag.pdf) DZKF 9/10-2012, DOP-THEMA-GYNÄMOLOGIE.
12. Kraft U., "Dem Diabetes auf die Spur. Ursprung des Diabetes Typ-1", Diabetes, no.2 (2016), pp 42–50.
13. Lee, H.S. et al., "Next-generation sequencing for viruses in children with rapid-onset type 1 diabetes", Diabetologia, 56 (8) Aug 2013, pp 1705–11, PMID 23657799.
14. Hettiarachi, K.D. et al., "The effects of repeated exposure to sub-toxic doses of plecomacrolide antibiotics on the endocrine pancreas", Food and chemical toxicology, 44(12) Dec 2006, pp 1966–77, PMID 16905235.
15. Arch Dis Child 93 2008 p 512, cited in Deutsche Ärzte Zeitung 3.3.2010 p 1, Leitartikel.
16. Beyerlein, A. et al., "Respiratory infections in early life and the development of islet autoimmunity in children at increased type I diabetes risk: evidence from the BABYDIET study", JAMA pediatrics, 167(9) Sept 2013, pp 800–807, PMID 23818010.
17. Kolb, H., "Kuhmilch und Diabetes", Monatszeitschrift für Kinderheilkunde, 149(13), 2001, pp 62–65.
18. Marietta, E.V. et al., "Low incidence of spontaneous type I diabetes in non-obese diabetic mice raised on gluten-free diets is associated with changes in the intestinal microbiome", PloS one, vol 8(11), 2013 S.e78687, doi: 10.1371/journal. pone.0078687, PMID 24236037.

19 Versorgungsleitlinien.de (http://www.versorgungs leitlinien.de/themen).
20 Yang, Q. et al., "Serum retinol binding protein 4 contributes to insulin resistance in obesity and type 2 diabetes", Nature, 436(7049), July 2005, pp 356–62, PMID 16034410.
21 Murki, I. et al., "Fruit consumption and risk of type 2 diabetes: results from three prospective longitudinal cohort studies", BMJ Clinical research, vol 347, 2013, p 5001, PMID 23990623.
22 Ling, W. et al., "Parental Psychological Stress reprograms haptic cluconeogensis in offspring" (http:// www.cell.com/cell-metabolism/fulltext/ S1550-4131(16)30006-7), Cell metabolism, doi: 10.1016/j.cmet.2016.01.014 (https://dx.doi.org/ 10.1016 %2Fj.cmet.2016.01.014).
23 Parker, J. et al., "Levels of vitamin D and cardiometabolic disorders: systematic review and meta-analysis", Maturitas, vol 65(3), March 2010, pp 225–36, PMID 20031348.
24 Stuebe, A.M. et al., "Duration of lactation and incidence of type 2 diabetes", JAMA, 294(20), Nov 2005, pp 2601–2610, PMID 16304074.
25 Jenkins, D.J. et al., "Glycemic index overview of implications in health and disease", Am J Clin Nutr, 2002(76), pp 266–273.
26 Salmeron, J. et al., "Dietary fiber, glycemic load, and risk of non-insulin-dependent diabetes mellitus in women", JAMA, 1997 (227), pp 472–77.
27 Salmeron, J., "Dietary fiber, glycemic load, and risk of NIDDM in men", Care, 1997, pp 20545–50.
28 Liu, S. et al., "A prospective study of dietary glycemic load and risk of myocardial infarction in women", Am J clin Nutr, 2000, 71, pp 1455–61.
29 Jeppersen, J. et al., "Effect of low-fat, high carbohydrate diets on risk factors for ischemic heart disease in postmenopausal women", Am J Clin Nutr, 1997, 65, pp 1027–33.
30 Liu, S. et al., "A prospective study of dietary fiber and risk of cardiovascular disease among women", Am J Coll Cardiol, 2002, 39, pp 49–56.
31 Rimm, E.B. et al., "Vegetable, fruit and dietary fiber intake and risk of coronary heart disease among men", JAMA, 1996, 275, pp 447–51.
32 Pietinen, P. et al., "Intake of dietary fiber and coronary heart disease in a cohort of Finnish men", Alpha tocopherol, Beta-Caroten Cancer Prevention Study, Circulation, 1996, 94, pp 2720–27.
33 Wolk, A.A. et al., "Long term intake of dietary fiber and decreased risk of coronary heart disease among women", JAMA 1999, 281, pp 1998–2004.
34 Jacobs, D.R. et al., "Fiber from whole grains, but not refined grains, is inversely associated with all-cause mortality in older women: the JOWA women's-health study", J Am Coll Nutr, 2000, 19 (3 suppl), 236, pp 129–33.
35 Gesundheitsbericht Deutschlands am Weltdiabetestag, 2016 https://www.deutsche-diabetes-gesellschaft.de/presse/ddg-pressemeldungen, viewed on 18 Dec 2017.
36 Gesundheitsbericht Deutschlands am Weltdiabetestag, 2010, http//www.diabetesorg.de, viewed on 18 Dec 2017.
37 Marx N., "Pathophysiologie der Arteriosklerose bei Diabetes mellitus", Clinical Research in Cardiology Supplements, Jan 2006.
38 Maahs, D.M. et al., "Hypertension prevalence, awareness, treatment, and control in an adult type diabetes Type 1 diabetes population and a comparable general population", Diabetes Care, 2005, 28, pp 301–6.
39 Grehn, F., Augenheilkunde, 30, published Heidelberg 2008, 217–22.
40 Kanski, J., Klinische Ophthalmologie, 6, published München, 2008, pp 581–99.
41 Aris, N. et al., "Diabetische Retinopathie", Deutsches Ärzteblatt, 107, (5) 2010, pp 75–84.
42 Nasemann, J., "Netzhaut (Retina)" in Sachsenweger, M., Duale Augenheilkunde, Stuttgart 2003, pp 259–62.
43 Nentwich, M.M. et al., "Diabetische Retinopathie" in Der Diabetologe, (6) 2010, pp 491 ff., Springer-Verlag.
44 Kook, D. et al., "Long-term effect of intravitreal bevacizumab (avastin) in patients with chronic diffuse diabetic macular edema", Retina, 2008, Oct 28 (8), pp 1053–60, PMID 18779710.
45 Kook, D. et al., "Long-term effect of intravitreal bevacinumab (avastin) in patients with chronic diffuse diabetic macular edema", Retina, 2008 (8), pp 1053–60, PMID 18779710.
46 Hakroush, S. et al., "Effects of increased renal tubular vascular endothelial growth factor (VEGF) on fibrosis, cyst formation, and glomerular disease", Am j of pathology, 175(5) m, 2009 m, pp 1883–95.

47 Juan, F. et al., "The role of inflammatory cytokines in diabetic nephropathy", J of the am society of nephrology: JASN", vol 19(3), March 2008, ISSN 15333450, PMID 18256353.
48 Freedman, B.I. et al., "Genetic factors in diabetic nephropathy", Clin J A,m Soc Nephrol, 2 2007, pp 1306–16.
49 Reddy, V.P. et al., "A versatile antioxydant and antiglycating agent", Science of Aging Knowledge Environment, 2005 (18), S. pe 12, PMID 15872311.
50 Imran, R. et al., "Carnosine and its constituents inhibit glycation of low density lipoproteins that promotes foam-cell formation in vitro", FEBS Letters, 581, (5) 2007, pp 1067–70.
51 Barry, I. et al., "Genetic factors in diabetic nephropathy", doi: 10.2215/CJN.02560607, CJASN, Nov 2007, vol 2, no 6, pp 1306–16.
52 Adler, et al., "Development and progression of nephropathy in type 2 diabetes: The United Kingdom Prospective Diabetes Study", in The Kidney Int., 2003, 63, p 225.
53 Richard, J.M. et al., "Nonalbuminuric renal insufficiency in type 2 diabetes", Diabetes care, vol 27(1), Jan 2004, ISSN 0149-5992.
54 Redaktion Deutsche Ärztezeitung: "The prevalence of gestational diabetes", 16 June 2017, doi: 10.3238 aerztebl.2017.0412 (https://dx.doi.org/10.3238%) (www.arztebl.de/10.3238/arztebl.2017.0412), viewed June 2017.
55 DGG, Deutsche Diabetesgesellschaft: "S-3 Leitlinie Gestationsdiabetes mellitus (GDM), Diagnostik, Therapie und Nachsorge", AWMF online, 2011 (http//www.awmf.org/leitlinien/detail/ll/057-008.html).
56 Weiss, P. et al., "Der vernachlässigte Gestationsdiabetes: Risiken und Folgen", Geburtsh Frauenheilk, 1999, 59, pp 535–44.
57 Bergenstal, R. et al., "Safety of a hybrid closed-loop insulin delivery system in patients with type 1 diabetes", Jama, 2016, 316 (13), pp 1407–18.
58 Fischer, S., "Aktuelle leitliniengerechte Therapie des Diabetes mellitus", Ars Medici, 12 2007, pp 605–16.
59 Pfeiffer, A. et al., "Therapie des Diabetes Typ 2", Deutsches Ärzteblatt Int, 2014, 111(5), pp 69–82.
60 Stellungnahme des BdSN zur ADIB-Operation (http/www.diabetes-news.de/content bdsn-nimmt-stellung).
61 Eliasson, B. et al., "Cigarette smoking and diabetes mellitus", Progress in Cardiovascular Disease, 45, pp 405–13.
62 Bott, S. et al., "Impact of smoking on the metabolic action of subcutaneous regular insulin in type 2 diabetic patients", Hormone and Metabolic Research, 37, pp 445–49.
63 Rösen, P. et al., "The role of oxydative stress in the onset and progression of diabetes and its complications: a summary of a Congress Series sponsored by UNESCO-MCBN, the American Diabetes Association and the German diabetes society", Diabetes/Metabolism Research and Reviews, 17, pp 189–212.
64 Mandrup-Poulsen, T. et al., "Beta cell death and protection", Annals of the New York Academy of Sciences, 1005.
65 Orth, S.R. et al., "Effects of smoking on renal function in patients with type 1 and type 2 diabetes mellitus", Nephrology Dialysis Transplantation, 20, pp 2414–19.
66 Tenenbaum, A. et al., "Smoking and development of type 2 diabetes mellitus among middle-aged and elderly Japanese men and women", Am J of Epidemiology, 160, pp 158–62.
67 Sairenchi, T. et al., "Cigarette smoking and risk of type 2 diabetes mellitus among middle-aged and elderly Japanese men and women", Am J Epidem, 160, pp 158–62.
68 Chowdhury, P. et al., "Pathophysiological effects of nicotine on the pancreas", Proceedings of the Society for Experimental Biology and Medicine, 218, pp 168–73.
69 Tziomalos, K. et al., "Endocrine effects of tobacco smoking", Clinical Endocrinology, 61, 2004, pp 664–74.
70 Wannamethee, G. et al., "Smoking as a modifiable risk factor for diabetes type 2 diabetes in middle-aged men", Diabetes Care, 24, 2001 (24), pp 1590–95.
71 Zheng, Y. et al., "Global etiology and epidemiology of type 2 diabetes mellitus and its complications", Nat Rew Endocrinol, 2017 Dec 8, doi: 10.1038/nrendo.2017.152 (Epub ahead of print), PMID 29219149.

72 Bundesärztekammer, Arzneimittelkommission der deutschen Ärzteschaft, Deutsche Diabetes-gesellschaft et al., "Nationale Versorgungsleitlinie Diabetes Typ 2", Kurzfassung 1st edition 2002, corrected version 1 April 2003.
73 Lim, J. et al., "Association of alcohol drinking patterns with presence of impaired fasting glucose and diabetes mellitus among South Korean adults", J epidemiol, 2017 Oct 28, doi: 10.2188/jea. JE20170021, PMID 29093361.
74 Vaeth, P. A. et al., "Ethnicity and alcohol consumption among US adults with diabetes", Ann epidemiol, 2014, Oct 24 (10), pp 720–6.
75 Imamura, F. et al., "Confounding by dietary patterns of the inverse association between alcohol consumption and type 2 diabetes risk", Am J Epidemiol, 2009 July 1, 170 (1), pp 37–45, PMID 19429876.
76 Beulens, J.W. et al., "Estimating the mediating effect of different biomarkers on the relation of alcohol consumption with the risk of type 2 diabetes", Ann epidemiol, 2013, April 23 (4), pp 193–7, PMID 23375342.
77 Holbrook, T.L. et al., "A prospective population-based study of alcohol use and non-insulin-dependent diabetes mellitus", Am J Epidemiol, 1990, Nov, 132 (5), pp 902–9.
78 Kao W.H. et al., "Alcohol consumption and the risk of type 2 diabetes mellitus: atherosclerosis risk in communities study", Am J Epidemiol, 2001, Oct 15, 154 (8), pp 748–57.
79 Fan, A.Z. et al., "Lifetime alcohol drinking pattern is related to the prevalence of metabolic syndrome", The Western New York Health Study (WNYHS), Eur J epidemiol, 2006, 21(2), pp 129–38.
80 Perneger, T.V. et al., "Risk of end-stage renal disease associated with alcohol consumption", Am J Epidemiol, 1999 Dec 15, 150 (12), pp 1275–81, PMID 10604769.
81 Pereira, M.A. et al., "Coffee consumption and risk of type 2 diabetes mellitus: an 11-year prospective study of 28,812 postmenopausal women", Arch Intern Med, 2006 June 26, 166 (12), pp 1311–6.
82 Kwok, M.K. et al., "Habitual coffee consumption and risk of type 2 diabetes, ischemic heart disease, depression and Alzheimer's disease: a Mendelian randomization study", Sci Rep, 2016, Nov 15, 6, 36500, doi:10.1038/srep.36500, PMID 27845333.
83 Williams, P.T. et al., "Coffee intake and elevated cholesterol and apolipoptrotein B levels in men."
84 Phillips, N.R. et al., "Levels and interrelationship of serum and lipoprotein cholesterol and triglycerides: association with adiposity and the consumption of ethanol, tobacco and beverages containing caffeine", Arteriosclerosis, 1981, Jan–Feb, 1(1), pp 13–24.
85 Klatsky, A.L. et al., "Coffee use prior to myocardial infarction restudied: heavier intake may increase the risk", Am J epidemiol, 1990, Sept, 132(3), pp 479–88, PMID 2389752.
86 Cowan, T.E. et al., "Chronic coffee consumption in the diet-induced obese rat: impact on gut microbiota and serum metabolites", J Nutr Biochem, 2014, April, 25(4), pp 489–95, PMID 24629912.
87 Bundesärztekammer, kassenärztliche Bundes-vereinigung, Arbeitsgemeinschaft der wissenschaft-lichen medizinischen Fachgesellschaften: Nationale Versorgungsleitlinie Therapie des Typ II Diabetes, 9 2013 Momento com, 8 April 2014 in internet archive (https://web.archive. Org/web/20140408225 426 (http://www.awmf.org/uploads 001gl S3 Typ II Diabetes_2013-09.pdf).
88 WHO BMI classification, Global Health Observatory (GHO), data 2008.
89 Bircher-Benner, M.O., Eine neue Ernährungslehre, Wendepunkt Verlag Berlin, Leipzig, Zürich, 10th edition, 1945.
90 Bircher-Benner, M.O., Grundzüge der Ernährungs-therapie auf Grund der Energie-Spannung der Nahrung. Verlag Otto Salle, Berlin, 1905 and 1905.
91 Kasnacev, V.P., in Jezowska-Trzebiatovska, B. et al., Photon emission from biological systems, proceedings of the first international Symposium, Wroclav, Poland, Jan. 1986.
92 Bischof, M., Biophotonen, das Licht in unseren Zellen, ISBN 3-86150-095-7.
93 Popp, F.A., Biologie des Lichtes, Grundlagen der ultraschwachen Zellstrahlung, Verlag Paul Parey, ISBN 3-489-61734-7.
94 Popp, F.A., Unsere Lebensmittel in neuer Sicht, ISBN 3-596-11459-4.
95 Van Vijck, R. and E., Utrecht University: "An Introduction to Human Biophoton Emission", Forsch Komplementärmed. Klass. Naturheilkd. 1005, 12, pp 77–83.
96 Prigogine, I. et al., Dialog mit der Natur, Piper Verlag München, ISBN 3-492-11181-5.

97 Pischinger, A., Das System der Grundregulation, Grundlagen für eine ganzheitsbiologische Theorie der Mediin, Huat-Verlag, Heidelberg, 1990. 8th expanded edition, ISBN: 3-7760-1183-1.
98 Chiasson, J.L.et al., "The STOP-NIDDM trial", JAMA, 2003, 290, pp 486-94.
99 Arznei-Telegramm, 2003, 34, pp 73 – 4.
100 Haffner, S.M. et al., "Effect of rosiglitazone treatment on non-traditional markers of cardiovascular disease in patients with type 2 diabetes mellitus", Circulation, 2002, 106(6), pp 679 – 84.
101 Bajaj, M. et al., "Decrease plasma adiponecrin concentrations are closely related to hepatic fat content and hepatic insulin resistance in pioglitazone-treated type 2 diabetic patients", J Clin endocrine Metab, 2004, 53, pp 2169 – 76.
102 Tiikkainen, M. et al., "Effects of rosiglitazone and metformin on liver fat content, hepatic insulin resistance, insulin clearance and gene expression in adipose tissue in patients with type 2 diabetes", Diabetes, 2004, 53, pp 2169 – 76.
103 Malmberg, K. et al., "Intense metabolic control by means of insulin in patients with diabetes mellitus and acute myocardial infarction (DIGAMI2): effects on mortality and morbidity", Eur Heart J, 2005, 26 (7), pp 650 – 61.
104 Amiel, S. A. et al., "Hypoglycaemia in type 2 diabetes", in Diabetic medicine: a journal of the British diabetic Association, vol 25(3), March 2008, pp 245 – 54, PMID 18215172.
105 Jezowska-Trzebiatowska et al., "Photon emission from biological systems, proceedings of the first international Symposium", Wroclav, Pland Jan, in Popp, F.A., Biologie des Lichtes, Grundlagen der ultraschwachen Zellstrahlung, Paul Parey-Verlag, ISBN 3-489 61734-7.
106 Bischof, M., Biophotonen: das Licht in unseren Zellen, Verlag 2001, ISBN 3-86150-095-7.
107 Van Vijck, R. et al., An Introduction to Human Biophoton Emission, Utrecht University Forsch. klass. Naturheilkunde, 1005, 12, pp 77 – 83.
108 Pischinger, A., Das System der Grundregulation, Grundlagen für eine ganzheitsbiologische Theorie der Medizin, Haug-Verlag Heidelberg, 1990, ISBN 3-7760-1183-1.
109 Bircher-Benner, M.O., Die Verhütung des Unheilbaren, Wendepunkt-Verlag Zürich, Leipzig, Wien, 2nd edition, vol 58.
110 Kollenbach, D., Bircher-Brenner, Maximilian Oskar (1867 – 1939), dissertation, Verlag der Medizinischen Fakultät der Universität Köln, 1974.
111 Losada, E. et al., "Real-world antidiabetic drug use and fracture risk in 12,277 patients with type 2 diabetes mellitus: a nested case-control study", Osteoporos Int., 2018 Jun 2, doi: 10.1007/s00198-018-4581-y, Epub ahead of print.
112 Wenzlau, J.M. dg yl., "The cation efflux transporter ZnT8 (Slc30A8) is a major autoantigen in human type 1 diabetes", PNAS 104, 17040 – 17045, 2007.
113 Sanjeevi, N. et al., "Trace element status in type 2 diabetes: a meta-analysis", J Clin Diagn Res., 2018 May, 12(5), OE01-OE08, doi: 10.7860/JCDR/2018/35026.11541.
114 Fernández-Cao, J.C. et al., "Dietary zinc intake and whole blood zinc concentration in subjects with type 2 diabetes versus healthy subjects: a systematic review, meta-analysis and meta-regression", J Trace Elem Med Biol., 2018 Sept, 49, pp 241 – 251, doi: 10.1016/j.jtemb.2018.02.008, Epub 2018 Feb 7.
115 Xyang, Y. et al., "Glutamic acid decarboxylase autoantibodies are dominant but insufficient to identify most Chinese with adult-onset non-insulin requiring autoimmune diabetes", LADA China study 5, Acta Diabetol, 2015 Dec, 52(6), pp1121 – 7, doi: 10.1007/s00592-015-0799-8, Epub 2015 Aug 5.
116 Leigh Broadhurst, C. et al.: "Clinical Studies on Chromium Picolinate Supplementation in Diabetes Mellitus, A Review", Diabetes Technology & Therapeutics, vol 8, no 6, review: http://doi.org/10.1089/dia.2006.8.677.
117 Liu, X.N. et al., "Effect of health literacy and exercise focused interventions on glycemic control in patients with type 2 diabetes in China", Abstract available in Chinese from the publisher, 2018, March 10 39(3), pp 357 – 62, doi:10.3760cma.j.issn0254 6450 2018.03.021.
118 Poblete-Aro C. et al.: Exercise and oxydatives stress in type 2 diabetes mellitus. Rev Med Chil. 2018 Mar;146(3):362-372. doi: 10.4067/s0034-98872018000300362. Spanish. PMID: 29999107.
119 Szilágyi, B. et al, "Sports therapy and recreation exercise program in type 2 diabetes: randomized controlled trial, 3-month follow-up", J Sports Med

Phys Fitness, 2018 July 9, doi: 10.23736/S0022-4707.18.08591-2, Epub ahead of print, PMID 29991214.
120 Gorres-Martens, B.K. et al., "Exercise prevents HFD- and OVX-induced type 2 diabetes risk factors by decreasing fat storage and improving fuel utilization", Physiol Rep, 2018, July, 6(13), e13783, doi: 10.14814/phy2.13783.
121 Belitz, H.D. et al., Lehrbuch der Lebensmittel-chemie, Springer, Berlin; 6th fully revised edition 2008, ISBN 978-3-540-73201-3, pp. 842–49.
122 Ido, Y. et al., "Interactions between the sorbitol pathway, non-enzymatic glycation, and diabetic vascular dysfunction", Nephrol Dial Transplant, 1996, 11 Suppl 5, pp 72–5.
123 Kajal, A. et al., "Modulation of Advanced Glycation End Products, Sorbitol, and Aldose Reductase by Hydroalcohol Extract of Lagenaria siceraria Mol Standl in Diabetic Complications: An In Vitro Approach", J Diet Suppl., 2018, July 4, 15(4), pp 482–498, doi: 10.1080/19390211.2017.1356419, Epub 2017 Sep 28.

Keyword index

3-deoxyglucone	28	antidiabetics, insulinotropic	62
ß-amyloid plaques	34	antidiabetics, non-insulinotropic	61
β-2 receptor	16	antioxidative substance	
β-cells	21, 23	provided by the body	33
β oxidation	16	ants, crawling	11
γ-proteins (TAU proteins)	34	apoplexy (stroke) and diebetes	31
abdominal pain	22	apoptosis (programmed cell death)	34
abscesses	11	appetite, loss of	11
A-cells	14	arsenic	35
acetic acid	21	arteriosclerosis and diabetes	25, 28, **31**, 67
acetone, acetone smell	11, **17**, **21**	arthritis	67
acetylcholine	29	artichokes, glycokine-like effect	70
acrylamide	28	autoantibodies against the	
actin phagocytosis	40	zinc transporter ZnT8	69
acupuncture	66	autoimmune reactions	19, 20, 35, 67
adhesion of the monocytes	29	autoimmune vasculitis	35
adipokines	30	badly healing wounds	31
adiponectin	40	Badsedow's inflammation	67
adrenalin	14, 16, 24	bafilomycin 1	20
aging process, premature	33	bafilomycin A 1	20
albumin	40	bafilomycins and diabetes typ 1	20
alcohol and diabetes	35, **53**, 56, 69	basal rate profile	49
aldehydes (α-β-unsaturated)	40	basal supported oral therapy (BOT)	48
alertness	21	basic regulation system	**65**
alpha glucosidase inhibitors	61	basis-bolus principle	49
Alzheimer's disease (AD)	10, 28, 34, 67	B-cells	14
amino acids	16	bean shell extract	69
amount of the amniotic fluid	42	beta folding sheet structure	34
amputations because diabetes	27	beta-hydroxybutyric acid	21
amylase inhibitors	68	biguanides	69
amyloids, amyloidosis	10, 35, 67	biological information	65
amyotrophic lateral sclerosis (ALS)	34	Bircher-Benner Diabetes Diet	**82**
analogue insulin glargine	45	Bircher-Benner diet, principles of the	75
analogue insulins	44	bitter melon	70
angina pectoris	11	bleeding into the vitreous body	37
annex and tables for the diabetes diet	123	blindness	27, **36**
antibiotics and typ 1 dieabetes	20	blood-brain barrier	11
antibodies against islet cells	20	blood fats, oxidised	36
antidiabetic bypass (ADIB)	52	blood glucose level, regulation of the	**14**
antidiabetics	43	blood pressure	29
antidiabetics (diabetes medicines)	**61**	blood-retina barrier	36

blood-sugar instability	11	cotton-wool spots	36
blood sugar level, correction of	**16**	coxsackie B virus	20
blood sugar level, fasting	11, 16	cramps in the calves	22
blueberry leaf tea	70	creatinine-albumin quotient	40
blue or pale discolouration of the toes	11	creatinine clearance	40
body mass index (BMI)	56	cross-reaction	20
body training	**76**	CTLA S4	19
bolus calculator	50	cytochrome C	34
bolus option	50	cytochrome P 450-oxidase	33
bread unit	82	cytomegalovirus (CMV)	20
brittle diabetes	48	D-cells	14
bromide radical (Br)	34	degeneration	17
cabbage	70	dehydration	21
cadmium	35	dementia	33
Caesarean section	20	dendritic cells	20
calcium	68	deoxyribonucleic acid (DNA)	64
cancer	33, 67	Desserts	119
carbohydrates	12, **24**, 82	detoxification enzyme	33
cardiovascular diseases	24, 26, **27**, 28, 31	diabetes criteria for children	12
		diabetes criteria of the WHO	12
carnosine	40	diabetes, gestational	**42**, 43
carnosine 1 gene	40	diabetes honeymoon	48
catalase	33	diabetes, rare types of	18
cataracts	38	diabetes typ 2, accepted partial causes	23
causes of type 1 diabetes	19	diabetes, type 1	18, **19**
celery	70	diabetes, type 2	18, **23**
cereal dishes	112	diabetes type 2, genetic risk factors for	24
chaperones	34	diabetic coma	21
charantin	70	diabetic foot syndrome	27, **31**
charcot foot	32	diabetic maculopathy	38
chemotherapy	35	diabetic nephropathy	10, **39**
chicory root	70	diabetic nephropathy, risk factors for	40
chloride radical (CI)	34	diabetic nephropathy with renal insufficiency	27
chlorophyll α-molecules	64		
cholesterol	10, **25**, 36, 67	diabetic neuropathy	10, 31
chromium	69	diabetic neuropathy (nerve degeneration)	27
cinquefoil (Potentilla aurea)	70		
civilisation diseases	66	diabetic polyneuropathy	28, **35**
clouding of consciousness	11	diabetic retinopathy	31, **36**
coagulation of the blood	29	diabetic retinopathy (retinal degeneration)	27
coenzyme Q10	33		
coffee and diabetes	54	diacylglycol	29
coherence	64	dialysis treatment	39, 41
coherence principle	65	dicarbonyl	28
colouring	27	dietary fibres	68
conventional insulin therapy (CT)	46	difficulty focusing	22
copalchi (Coutarea latifolia)	70	disease	65
copper	35, 69	disposable insulin syringes	46
cortisol	14, 16, 24, 42	dissipative system	65

DNA peroxidation	33	general directives for order therapy	
drowsiness	11	for diabetes	**71**
ductus pancreaticus	14	genes HLA-A	19
echo viruses	20	genes HLA-B	19
electrolyte shifts	21	genetic polymorphism	40, 54
electromagnetic radiation	33	gestational diabetes	**42**
endocrine pancreas	14	glaucoma	10, 67
endogenous glycation	28	glinides	62
endothelial dysfunction	**29**, 31, 39	glitazone	61
endothelin-1 (ET-1)	29	glomeruli	39, 67
energy: orderly and chaotic	64	glucagon	14, 16, 24
enterohepatic circulation	66	gluconeogenesis	16, 21, 24
epidemic diabetes	9	glucose	11, 28, 39
epigenetic mutation	24	glucose level	11, 13
essential oil	26	glucose level, correction of	**15**
excessive urine (Polyurie)	11	glucose tolerance test	**13**, 42
excretion of urine (polyuria)	17	glucose transporters GLUT1	39
exocrine pancreas	14	glucose transport proteins of type 4	
exogenous glycation	27	(GLUT 4	23
exsiccosis	21	GLUT-4 receptors	18, 23
eyesight problems	11	glutamate	34
fat metabolism	26	glutathione	33
fat-soluble flavones	70	glutathione reductase	33
fatty acids	16, 17, 21, 33	gluten exposure	21
fatty liver	66	glycaemic charge	**26**, 138
fatty streaks	67	glycaemic index (GI)	**26**, 28, 67, 138
feeling of paralysis	11	glycation	**27**, 28, 31, 33,
ferritin	69		38, 39, 40, 72
fibrinolysis	29	glycation end products (AGEs)	27, 32
fibronectin	30	glycogen	15
flavours	27	glycogen phosphorylase (PYG)	16
flood of uric acid (gout)	71	glycogen synthase (GYS)	15
flow-shearing forces	29	glycohemoglobin (HbA1c)	13, 36
foam cells	31	glycokines	69, 70
folia orthosiphonis	70	golden-yellow	70
food energy	**64**	growth factors	36
forms of insulin therapy	**46**	guanine	69
free radicals	29, **33**	haemoglobin A1C	28
frequency	19	haemorrhoids	66
Fresh juices	90	hardening of the vascular walls	30
fresh plant-based	72	hard exudates	36
fresh vegetable foods	65	harms the large blood vessels	
fructose	25, 28, 39, **72**	(macroangiopathy)	31
fructose (also called laevulose)	72	HbA1c	12
fruit juices	23	headache	22
functional insulin therapy (FIT)	47	heart attack	26, 27, 31, 67
galactose	28, 39	heme oxygenase-1 (HO-1)	24
galega (galea officinalis)	69	herpes viruses	20
galegin	69	high blood pressure	31

high blood pressure, fixated	30	insulin therapy for type 2 diabetes	48, 62
human placental lactogen	42	insulin, types of	**44**
hungry	17	insulitis	21
Huntington's disease	34	integral law of nutrition	67
hyaline	39	intensified conventional	
hybrid closed loop system	49	insulin therapy (ICT)	46
hydrogen peroxide (H2O2)	33	intercapillary glomerulonephritis	39
hydroxide radical (OH)	33	intercellular substance (matrix)	25, **65**
hydroxyl radical (OH)	34	interleukin 1	28
hygiene	77	interleukin-1α, 6, 18 and TNF α	39
hyperglycaemia	29	interleukins	16
hyperinsulinism	18, **23**	Intermediate-acting insulins	45
hypersensitivity to light	35	intestinal flora	20, 66
hypertension	27, 36, 42	intestine	35
hypoglycaemia	42, **63**	iron	69
hypohidrosis	35	islet cells of the pancreas	**14**
hypophysis	16	islets of Langerhans	14
ideal weight	57	Itching	11
Illness	24	Jerusalem artichokes	70
immune competence	66	ketoacidosis	**17**, 21
immunocompetence	19	ketone bodies	17
impotence	35	ketonic acid flood	72
inexplicable blood sugar fluctuations	48	kidney	31
infants	20	kidney failure	67
infections	35	kidney tea (Koemis Koetjing)	69
inflammation mediators	16	Kimmelstiel-Wilson syndrome	39
inflammation of the urinary tract	42	Koemis Koetjing (kidney tea)	69
inflammation readiness	30	lack of movement	24
inflammatory cytokines	39	lactation	21
information	**65**, 67	Lactation	24
injections into the vitreous body	38	lactose	25
inner layer of the blood vessels (endothelium)	29	laminin	30
		Langerhans	20, 23
INS	19	laser amplification	64
insulin	14, **15**, 26	laser threshold	64
insulin deficit	21	laser treatment of the retina	38
insulin injection, methods of	45	LDL cholesterol	25, **31**
insulin level	27	LDL molecule	67
insulin-like growth factor	28	lead	35
insulin pen	46	lectins	68
insulin pumps	50	leg cramps	11
insulin resistance	**23**, 24, 27, 41, 42	lemons	70
		lente insulins	45
insulin, resistant to	9	leptin	40
insulin signal path	30	lettuce	70
insulin therapy	48	Lewy bodies	34
Insulin therapy	**44**	life order and body training	76
insulin therapy at shift work or irregular daily rhythm	47	lipid peroxidation	33, 34
		living raw plant food	65

lung emphysema (COPD)	28	non-proliferative retinopathy	36
macroalbuminuria	40	NO-synthase	34
macrophages	31	NPH insulins	45
macula degeneration	**38**	nutritive stimulus	68
macular degeneration	10, 67	oats	70
maculopathy	38	obesity	18, 23, 26, 30, 31, 42, 52
magnesium	69		
malformations	42	obesity, assessment of body weight	56
matrix	**65**	oestrogens	42
matrix (intercellular substance)	**25**	oranges	70
medication	68	order therapy for diabetes mellitus	**64**
medicinal herbs for treating diabetes	**69**	osteoporosis	28, 67, 69
medicines	35	over-acidification with keto bodies	68
mental health issues	75	oxidation	17
mercury	35	oxygen deficit	29
metabolic slags	66	pancreas	**14**
metabolic syndrome	24	pancreatic polypeptide	14
metformin	61	paralysis	35
methods of insulin injection	45	paraneoplastic syndrome	35
methylglyoxal	28	peripherally caused atactic coordination issues	35
MHC region	19		
microalbuminuria	40, 41	peripheral vascular disease (PVD)	27
microaneurysms	36	peroxidation of unsaturated fatty acids	40
microangiopathy	31, 36, 39	peroxide dismutase	33
mineral metabolism	**68**	peroxynitrite	34
miscarriages	42	peroxynitrite (ONOO-)	30
mitochondria	25, 33	Peyer's patches	19
mixed insulins	45	phenotypical polymorphism	40
molecular mimicry	20	phosphate	68
monocytes	28	photons	64, 67
movement	70, 75	photon storage	65
moving	52	phytic acid	68
multiple sclerosis (MS)	34	phytochemicals	67
multiple vaccinations	21	p-insulin	70
myelin	28	plant-based fresh foods (raw food)	67
NADPH oxydase	29	plant milk types	90
nephropathy	36	plant substances, secondary	26, 33, 67
nephropathy, diabetic	10, 39, 43	plant substances, secondary (phytochemicals)	68
nephrosis	67		
nerve conduction speed	35	plasminogen activator 1 (PAI-1 and ET-1)	30
neurodegenerative diseases	**33**		
neuropathy	34, 35	platelet-derived growth factor	28
neuropathy, diabetic	10, 31	polydipsia	21
nitric oxide (NO)	33	polydipsia (thirst)	42
nitrogen monoxide (NO)	29, 30	Polydipsie (increased thirst)	11
nitrogen oxide radical (NO)	34	polymorphism	40
NMDA receptor	34	polyneuropathy	32
NO	34	polyphenols	68
nodular glomerulosclerosis	39	polyurie (excessive urine)	11, 21

potassium	68		roasting	28
potato dishes	109		rot toxins	66
PP-cells	14		rowan	72
pregnancy	13, 17, 36, 37		rubella infection	20
Pregnancy with diabetic nephropathy	43		rubeosis iridis	37
principle of chaos	65		rubeotic secondary glaucoma	37
problem of food energy	59		saccharose	25
problems emptying	35		secondary diseases	27
progesterone	42		selenium	33, 69
prolactin	42		Semilente insulins	45
proliferative retinopathy	36		Sensor-supported pump therapy (SuP)	50
protease inhibitors	68		sensory impairment	35
protein C	39		sepsis	28
protein kinase C (PKC)	29		short summary	80
protein peroxidation	33		Signs of acute danger	11
pseudo normalisation	41		Silubin	69
psychological support	78		sleep before midnight	41
PTPN1 gene	24		somatostatin	14
puberty	36, 37		soups	92
quantity of food	73		spa stays	70
quitting smoking as part of the			stages of diabetic nephropathy	41
basic treatment for diabetes	52		standard value of the	
radical captors	40		blood glucose level	12
radical scavengers	40		stinging nettle	70
reaction of the synthetic insulin	22		stress and type 2 diabetes	24
reactive oxidising substances (ROS)	40		stress axis	16
reactive oxygen species (ROS)	29, **33**, 34		stress, electromagnetic	41
readiness for inflammation	16		stress on the blood glucose level	16
recipe section	84		stress, oxidative	17, 28, 30, 31, 33, 40
recipe section, fats and oils	91			
recipes for fresh plant-based foods			stress, physical	24
(raw food)	84		strictly thermal food energy	
regime for intensified insulin therapy	51		in kilocalories	59
regular insulin	44		stroke	27, 67
renal insufficiency	40		sugar in the diet	83
replacement products made			sulfonyl-urea derivatives	62
of cow's milk	21		sunflowers	70
re-resorption capacity of the kidneys	17		sunlight	64, 67
respiratory chain of the mitochondria	33		superfine flour	24, 26
respiratory infections in childhood			superoxide anion radical (O_2^-)	**33**
and type 1 diabetes	20		supplementary insulin therapy (SIT)	47
retinal infarctions	36		surfen	45
retinal oedema	36		surgical treatment of	
retinol binding protein 4 (RBP-4)	23		diabetic retinopathy	38
retinopathy	10		sympathicus	16
rheumatism medicines	69		synovial layer of the joints	67
rheumatism (polyarthritis)	28		system of lymph vessels	66
risk factors	42		Syzygium jambolana tree	70
risk factors for diabetic nephropathy	40		tannins	68

Teas	121	VEGF (vascular endothelial growth factor)	39
TGF-β (tissue growth factor β)	39		
thallium	35	vibrancy of food	67
therapy protocol	47	viruses as a partial cause of type 1 diabetes	20
thermodynamics	59, 60, 65		
thirst, increased (Polydipsie)	11, 17, 42	vitamin A	33
thorny burnet	70	vitamin B1	35
tractive retinal detachment	37	vitamin B12	35, 67
treatment of type 2 diabetes	52, **55**	vitamin C	33
treatment targets	51	vitamin D	20, 24
treatment with the insulin pump	48	vitamin E	33, 35
triglyceride blood level	31	vomiting	21
triglyceride levels	26, 36	warning signs for diabetes	11
tumour necrosis factor α (TNF-α)	30	water applications	77
tyrosine-phosphatase (N1)	24	weight loss	**21**
ubiquinone	33	Weight loss	11
vanadium	69	WHO	18
varicose veins	67	wholemeal	26
vasoconstriction	29	wound healing	28
vasodilatation	29	zinc	45, 68
vegetables	96		

CENTRE FOR SCIENTIFIC NATURAL MEDICINE

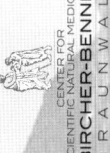

People come to the Bircher-Benner Medical Centre from a large number of countries in search of healing.

Here, you will be valued as a unique person, listened to and understood. Here, humanity and dignity are important and the medicine is a noble undertaking.

The search for the true causes of diseases is central to our work, as is the inclusion of your self-curative powers in the process of healing.

Centre for scientific natural medicine

Our fresh-vegetable diet will bring about a rapid change in your metabolism; natural regulative therapies take precedence where possible.

The atmosphere and the living tradition of the Bircher-Benner Centre, where novelty and modernity are combined with decades of experience, contribute to your healing.

The doctors and therapists will treat you personally and have all the facilities of a modern clinic at hand when needed.

The supplementation of traditional medicine by the regulative diagnosis and therapy of natural healing often permits a cure where the usual therapies have failed.

In the Medical Centre, you can relax and recover, and will experience the deep regeneration of your healing powers.

CENTRE BIRCHER-BENNER
CH-8784 Braunwald

Phone: +41 (0)21 801 60 04
Fax: +41 (0)55 643 16 93
info@bircher-benner.com
www.bircher-benner.com

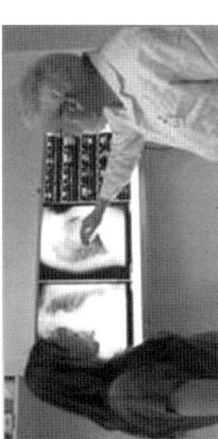

Indications: any internal diseases, migraine, tinnitus, neuralgia and other pain conditions, fibromyalgia, arthritis and arthrosis, collagenoses, liver, gallbladder and gastrointestinal diseases, metabolic diseases and diabetes, cardiovascular diseases, kidney and prostate diseases, women's diseases, allergies, skin diseases, convalescence, fatigue, depression and anxiety, menopausal, hormonal and weight problems.